IoT-Enabled Smart Healthcare Systems, Services and Applications

IoT-Enabled Smart Healthcare Systems, Services and Applications

Edited by

Shalli Rani
Chitkara University, Punjab, India

Maheswar Rajagopal
VIT Bhopal University, Bhopal, India

Neeraj Kumar
Thapar Institute of Engineering and Technology, Patiala, India

Syed Hassan Ahmed Shah
IEEE & ACM Senior Member

WILEY

This edition first published 2022

Registered Office
John Wiley & Sons, Inc., 111 River Street, Hoboken, NJ 07030, USA

Editorial Office
9600 Garsington Road, Oxford, OX4 2DQ, UK

For details of our global editorial offices, customer services, and more information about Wiley products visit us at www.wiley.com.

Wiley also publishes its books in a variety of electronic formats and by print-on-demand. Some content that appears in standard print versions of this book may not be available in other formats.

Library of Congress Cataloging-in-Publication Data

Names: Rani, Shalli, editor.
Title: Iot-enabled smart healthcare systems, services and applications / edited by Shalli Rani, Chitkara University, Punjab, India, Maheswar Rajagopal, VIT Bhopal University, Bhopal, India, Neeraj Kumar, Thapar Institute of Engineering and Technology, Patiala, India, Syed Hassan Ahmed Shah, IEEE & ACM Senior Member.
Description: Hoboken, NJ : Wiley, 2022. | Includes bibliographical references and index.
Identifiers: LCCN 2021038154 (print) | LCCN 2021038155 (ebook) | ISBN 9781119816799 (hardback) | ISBN 9781119816805 (adobe pdf) | ISBN 9781119816812 (epub)
Subjects: LCSH: Medical informatics.
Classification: LCC R118 .I58 2022 (print) | LCC R118 (ebook) | DDC 610.285–dc23
LC record available at https://lccn.loc.gov/2021038154
LC ebook record available at https://lccn.loc.gov/2021038155

Cover Design: Wiley
Cover Image: © everything possible/Shutterstock

Set in 9.5/12.5pt STIXTwoText by Straive, Pondicherry, India

10 9 8 7 6 5 4 3 2 1

MIX
Paper from responsible sources
FSC
www.fsc.org
FSC® C013604

Contents

Preface

This book presents various features of how smart healthcare can be used to analyze diseases, the underlying methodologies, and related security concerns. Healthcare is a multidisciplinary field that includes a range of aspects such as social issues, healthcare technologies, and healthcare frameworks, all of which affect the healthcare provided to individuals and families. The objectives of healthcare services include patients' security as well as treatment timeliness, effectiveness, and reliability. Smart healthcare comprises m-health, e-health, data transmission, smart and intelligent home services, medical devices, and so forth. The Internet of Things (IoT) is a system comprising real-world things that interact and communicate with each other via networking technologies. Nowadays, IoT is fully involved in the healthcare domain because it is suitable for remote health monitoring, it makes life easier and safer, it helps patients' rehabilitation, and so forth. Healthcare analytics can be used on the gathered data of heterogenous objects to improve healthcare at minimum expense, which is useful for healthcare experts.

In the emerging field of IoT and in the present worldwide scenario, there is a huge demand for healthcare services. It has evolved from the situations and conditions arising day by day to keep ourselves informed and aware of healthcare services. This book is going to attract and provide the platform to researchers, scholars, and industrialists to have an all-encompassing view of healthcare research We are looking forward to its enhancements and extensions as the healthcare services progression in IoT, which is quite obvious because the health domain is an ever-demanding area of research in services with the aid of technologies such as machine learning, image processing, data analytics, data gathering, cloud services, remote monitoring, and wireless communications. People will get one platform for architectures, services, use case scenarios, and data management, and this will enable them to formulate new research ideas. Advancements in machine learning, deep learning, cloud computing, and so forth, give a boost to the healthcare domain in the field of IoT. The book provides step-by-step guidance starting from the general knowledge and ending toward implementations in form of use case scenarios, and it will guide novice users to work on this domain.

Acknowledgments

First and foremost, I would like to thank my husband, **Shvet Jain,** for standing beside me throughout my research career so far and editing this book. He has been my motivation for continuing to improve my knowledge and move forward in my career. He is my lifetime achievement, and I dedicate this book of mine to him.

Moreover, without the prayers and best wishes of my parents, my sister, and both of my sons, none of my achievements would have been possible.

I am also thankful to the Wiley editorial team and my co-editors, **Dr. Neeraj Kumar, Dr. R. Maheswar, and Dr. Syed Hassan Ahmed Shah**, who really helped me in every aspect in the preparation of this book. Their prompt response and care to the literature and contribution is remarkable. They are great and responsible researchers indeed.

I would also like to thank each and every one behind the completion of this book, especially **Dr. Syed Hassan Ahmed Shah**, who actually helped a lot, and without his quick and efficient efforts, it wouldn't have been possible to get our book published. He motivated and gave me this platform to go ahead.

Last but not least, my gratitude is due to my inspiration **Dr. Archana Mantri**, Vice Chancellor, Chitkara University, Punjab, for her trust in me and for making me confident that I can put efforts to be successful in each and every field.

About the Editors

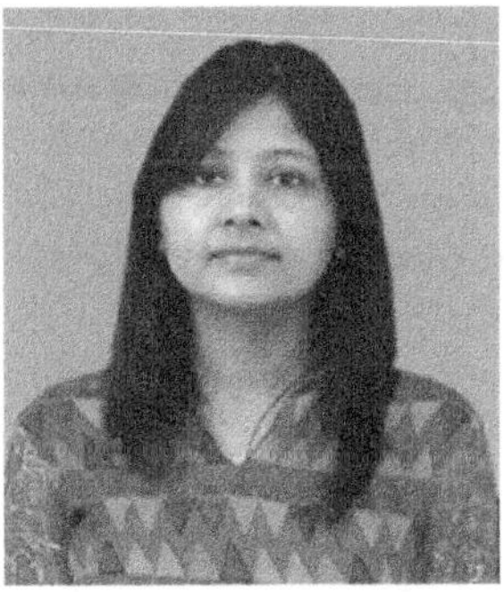

Dr. Shalli Rani (member IEEE) is associate professor in CSE with Chitkara University, Rajpura, Punjab, India. She has 15+ years of teaching experience. She received an MCA degree from Maharishi Dyanand University, Rohtak, in 2004, an M.Tech. degree in computer science from Janardan Rai Nagar Vidyapeeth University, Udaipur, in 2007, and a PhD degree in computer applications from Punjab Technical University, Jalandhar, in 2017. Her main areas of interest and research are wireless sensor networks, underwater sensor networks, and Internet of Things. She has published and presented more than 50 papers in international journals/conferences (SCI+Scopus) and two books with Springer. She is serving as an associate editor of IEEE *Future Directions Newsletter*. She has worked on big data, cloud computing, fog computing, underwater acoustic sensors, and IoT to show the importance of WSN in IoT applications. She won the Young Scientist Award in February 2014 from Punjab.

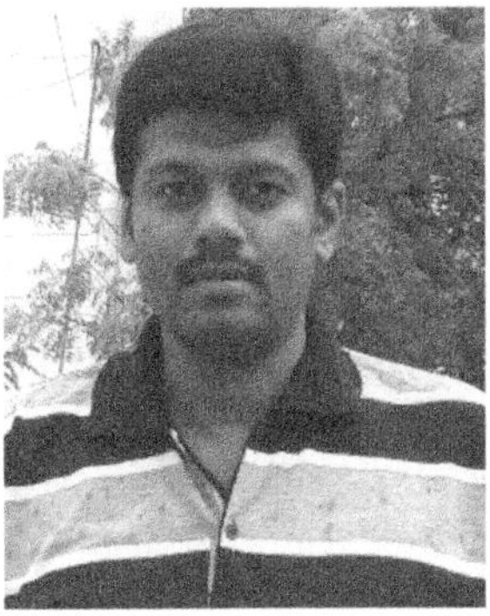

Dr. Maheswar Rajagopal has completed his B.E (ECE) from Madras University in 1999, and M.E (applied electronics) from Bharathiyar University in 2002, and a PhD in the field of wireless sensor networks from Anna University in 2012. He has about 19 years of teaching experience at various levels and is presently working as Dean – Research (Assistant) and Dean In-Charge for the School of EEE, VIT Bhopal University, Bhopal. He has published around 70 papers at international journals and international conferences and published four patents. His research interests include wireless sensor networks, IoT, queueing theory, and performance evaluation. He has served as guest editor for *Wireless Networks Journal*, Springer, currently serves as editorial review board member for peer-reviewed journals, and has also edited four books supported by EAI/Springer Innovations in Communications and Computing book series. He is presently an associate editor in the *Wireless Networks Journal*, Springer, *Alexandria Engineering Journal*, Elsevier, and *Ad-hoc Sensor Wireless Networks Journal*, Old City Publishing.

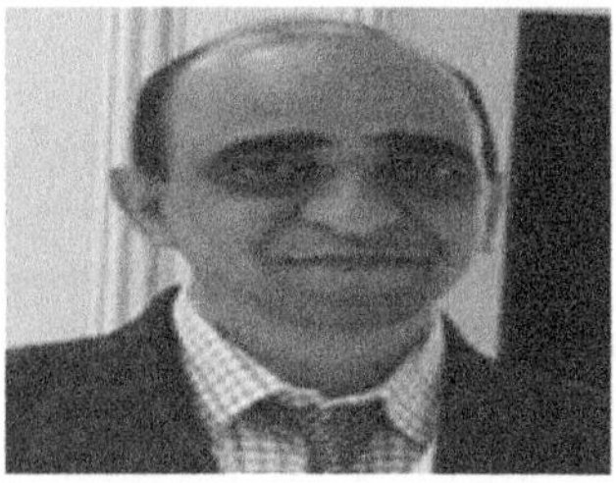

Professor Neeraj Kumar (SMIEEE) is a full professor in the Department of Computer Science and Engineering, Thapar Institute of Engineering and Technology, Patiala (Pb.), India. He is also adjunct professor at Asia University, Taiwan, King Abdul Aziz University, Jeddah, Saudi Arabia, and Charles Darwin University, Australia. He has published more than 400 technical research papers (DBLP: https://dblp.org/pers/hd/k/Kumar_0001:Neeraj) in top-cited journals and conferences, which have been cited more than 17000 times from well-known researchers across the globe, with current h-index of 71 (Google scholar: https://scholar.google.com/citations?hl=en&user=gL9gR-4AAAAJ). He was highly cited researcher in 2019 and 2020 in the list released by Web of Science (WoS). He has guided many research scholars leading to PhD and M.E./M.Tech degrees. His research is supported by funding from various competitive agencies across the globe. His broad research areas are green computing and network management, IoT, big data analytics, deep learning, and cybersecurity. He has also edited/authored 10 books with international and national publishers such as IET, Springer, Elsevier, CRC: *Security and Privacy of Electronic Healthcare Records: Concepts, Paradigms and Solutions* (ISBN-13: 978-1-78561-898-7), *Machine Learning for Cognitive IoT*, CRC Press, *Blockchain, Big Data and Machine Learning*, CRC Press, *Blockchain Technologies across Industrial Vertical*, Elsevier, *Multimedia Big Data Computing for IoT Applications: Concepts, Paradigms and Solutions* (ISBN: 978-981-13-8759-3), *Proceedings of First International Conference on Computing, Communications, and Cyber-Security* (IC4S 2019; ISBN 978-981-15-3369-3), and *Probabilistic Data Structures for Blockchain based IoT Applications*, CRC Press. One of the textbooks he edited, entitled *Multimedia Big Data Computing for IoT Applications: Concepts, Paradigms, and Solutions*, published in Springer in 2019, has had 3.5 million downloads as of June 2020. It attracts the attention of the researchers across the globe. (https://www.springer.com/in/book/9789811387586). He serves as editor of *ACM Computing Survey, IEEE Transactions on Sustainable Computing, IEEE Systems Journal, IEEE Network Magazine, IEEE Communication Magazine, Elsevier Journal of Networks and Computer Applications, Elsevier Computer Communication,* and *Wiley International Journal of Communication Systems.* Also, he has organized various special issues of journals of repute from IEEE, Elsevier, and Springer. He has been a workshop chair at IEEE Globecom 2018, IEEE Infocom 2020 (https://infocom2020.ieee-infocom.org/workshop-blockchain-secure-software-defined-networking-smart-communities) and IEEE ICC 2020 (https://icc2020.ieee-icc.org/workshop/ws-06-secsdn-secure-and-dependable-software-defined-networking-sustainable-smart) and Track Chair of Security and Privacy of IEEE MSN 2020 (https://conference.cs.cityu.edu.hk/msn2020/cf-wkpaper.php). He is also TPC Chair and member of various international conferences such as IEEE MASS 2020 and IEEE MSN2020. He has won the best papers award from *IEEE Systems* journal and IEEE ICC 2018, Kansas City, in 2018. He won the best researcher award from a parent organization every year for the last eight consecutive years.

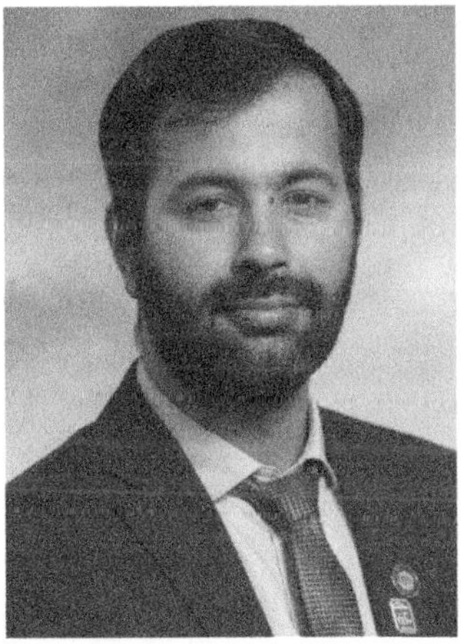

Dr. Syed Hassan Ahmed Shah (SM'18) Ahmed is IEEE Senior Member and ACM Distinguished Speaker. He currently works at JMA Wireless as a product specialist for distributed antenna systems (DAS), CBRS, small cell, and the virtualized RAN product line. Previously, he was an assistant professor in the Department of Computer Science at Georgia Southern University, US, where, he also founded the Wireless Internet and Networking Systems (WINS) lab. Prior to this, he was a Post-Doctoral Fellow in the Department of Electrical and Computer Engineering, University of Central Florida, Orlando, US. Before moving to the United States, he completed his BS with honors in CS from Kohat University of Science & Technology (KUST), Pakistan, and Master combined PhD degree from the School of Computer Science and Engineering (SCSE), Kyungpook National University (KNU), Republic of Korea (South Korea). In the summer of 2015, he was also a visiting researcher at Georgia Tech, Atlanta, US. Overall, he has authored/coauthored over

200 international publications including journal articles, conference proceedings, book chapters, and three books. In 2016, his work on robust content retrieval in future vehicular networks led him to win the Qualcomm Innovation Award at KNU, Korea. Dr. Hassan's research interests include sensor and ad hoc networks, cyber-physical systems, vehicular communications, and future Internet. He has been an appointee of the Board of Governors of the IEEE Vehicular Technology Society as liaison to IEEE Young Professionals society for 2018–2019. Since 2018, he is also an ACM Distinguished Speaker. Furthermore, Dr. Hassan is a Senior IEEE and ACM professional member, has served as a TPC Member or Reviewer in 100+ international conferences and workshops including IEEE Globecom, IEEE ICC, IEEE CCNC, IEEE ICNC, IEEE VTC, IEEE INFOCOM, ACM CoNEXT, ACM MobiHoc, and ACM SAC. Additionally, he has been reviewing papers for 30+ international journals including *IEEE Wireless Communications* magazine, networks, communications, *IEEE Communications Letters, IEEE Sensors Letters, IEEE Transactions on Industrial Informatics, Vehicular Technologies, Intelligent Transportation Systems, Big Data*, and *Mobile Computing*. Moreover, Dr. Hassan has been an editorial member of more than 30 special issues with top-ranked journals in Communication Society and has served as an editorial board member of KSII Transactions on Internet & Information Systems and Wiley's *Internet Technology Letters, Transactions on Emerging Telecommunications Technologies, IEEE Newsletters on Internet Initiative, Future Directions*, and *Software Defined Networks*.

List of Contributors

Masooma Zehra Syeda
Division of Nano & Information Technology
Center for Imaging Media Research, KIST(Korea Institute of Science and Technology)
Seoul
Republic of Korea

Dur-e-hassan Syeda
Department of Software Engineering
Mehran University of Engineering and Technology
Jamshoro
Sindh
Pakistan

Himanshi Babbar
Chitkara University Institute of Engineering and Technology
Chitkara University
Punjab
India

Divya Gupta
Chitkara University Institute of Engineering and Technology
Chitkara University
Punjab
India

Shalli Rani
Chitkara University Institute of Engineering and Technology
Chitkara University
Punjab
India

Syed Hassan Ahmed Shah
Product Specialist, JMA wireless
USA

Neeraj Kumar
Department of Computer Science and Engineering
Thapar University
Patiala
Punjab
India

R. Nidhya
Department of Computer Science and Engineering, Madanapalle Institute of Technology & Science
Madanapalle
Andhra Pradesh
India

Manish Kumar
School of Computer Science and Engineering
Vellore Institute of Technology
Chennai, Tamil Nadu
India

R. Maheswar
Dean Research (Assistant), VIT Bhopal University
Bhopal
India

D. Pavithra
Department of Electronics and Communication Engineering,
Sri Ramakrishna Institute of Technology
Coimbatore, Tamil Nadu
India

M. Saravanan
Department of Electronics and Communication Engineering, Sri Eshwar College of Engineering
Coimbatore, Tamilnadu, India

J. Ajayan
Department of Electronics and Communication Engineering, SR University
Warangal, Telangana
India

R. Maheswar
School of Electrical & Electronics Engineering (SEEE), VIT Bhopal University
Sehore
Madhya Pradesh
India

E. Parthasarathy
Department of Electronics and Communication Engineering, SRM Institute of Science and Technology
Chennai, Tamilnadu
India

Shanu Bhardwaj
Chitkara University Institute of Engineering and Technology
Chitkara University
Punjab
India

S.N. Panda
Chitkara University Institute of Engineering and Technology
Chitkara University
Punjab
India

Priyanka Datta
Chitkara University Institute of Engineering and Technology
Chitkara University
Punjab
India

Rajesh Kumar Kaushal
Chitkara University Institute of Engineering and Technology
Chitkara University
Punjab
India

Naveen Kumar
Chitkara University Institute of Engineering and Technology
Chitkara University
Punjab
India

Amit Sundas
School of Engineering, Ajeenkya
DY Patil University
Pune
India

Sumit Badotra
School of Computer Science &
Engineering, Faculty of Engineering
& Technology, Jain University
Karnataka
India

Chhabildas Madhukar Gajare
School of Engineering, Ajeenkya
DY Patil University
Pune
India

Chetna Kaushal
Chitkara University Institute of
Engineering and Technology
Chitkara University
Punjab
India

Md Khairul Islam
Department of Information and
Communication Technology
Islamic University, Kushtia
Bangladesh

Anshu Singla
Chitkara University Institute of
Engineering and Technology
Chitkara University
Punjab
India

Md Al Amin
Department of Computer Science
and Engineering
Prime University
Dhaka
Bangladesh

Ravneet Kaur
School of Information Technology
Deakin University
Victoria, Geelong
Australia
Chitkara University Institute
of Engineering and Technology
Chitkara University
Punjab
Rapura
India

Ramkumar Ketti Ramachandran
Chitkara University Institute of
Engineering and Technology
Chitkara University
Punjab, Rapura
India

Robin Doss
School of Information Technology
Deakin University
Victoria, Geelong
Australia

Lei Pan
School of Information Technology
Deakin University
Victoria, Geelong
Australia

1

The Role of Emerging Technologies in Smart Healthcare

Masooma Zehra Syeda[1], Dur-e-hassan Syeda[2], and Himanshi Babbar[3]

[1]*Division of Nano & Information Technology, Center for Imaging Media Research, KIST(Korea Institute of Science and Technology), Seoul, Republic of Korea*
[2]*Department of Software Engineering, Mehran University of Engineering and Technology, Jamshoro, Sindh, Pakistan*
[3]*Chitkara University Institute of Engineering and Technology, Chitkara University, Punjab, India*

1.1 Introduction

Environmental pollution is an important factor that affects the health of every age group. Health improvement is an urgent need to improve quality of life. Owing to the advancements in computation and communication technologies, the healthcare sector has benefited handsomely from the available tools and applications [1]. Healthcare-related actors (doctors, facilitators, practitioners, researchers, and strategic planners) are striving to address the challenges faced by the current healthcare system by continuously struggling with the healthcare system performance. Till date, a plethora of smart tools pertaining to electronic healthcare are used. It is important to note that the healthcare enhancements enable a positive change to become smart healthcare. Sufficient access to healthcare is related to an increment in life expectancy of about 2.0–2.5 years in men and women at age of 65 as reported in China [2]. Many of the research directions at the emergence of data analytics, wireless communication, information security, intelligent networks, and AI-equipped methods that provide early diagnosis, prevention, and constant treatment of health conditions. These new technologies and techniques are visualized as the basic elements of modern healthcare. Gunther Eysenbach indicated that healthcare is to be improved

IoT-Enabled Smart Healthcare Systems, Services and Applications, First Edition.
Edited by Shalli Rani, Maheswar Rajagopal, Neeraj Kumar and Syed Hassan Ahmed Shah.

worldwide and locally with the utilization of information and communication technology [2]. The deliverance of smart healthcare depends on groups of instructed caregivers and emerging technology mediums. Healthcare systems that are routinely used nowadays were not long ago just a vision beyond our technological frontier. Therefore, the emergence of technology and digital systems (consisting of many heterogeneous sensors and computing devices) has created a chance to transform traditional healthcare systems with Internet-based systems to harness the benefits of cutting-edge technologies. Smart healthcare leverages these new emerging technologies to transform the traditional medical measures. The patient will experience better care, and they are fundamentally changing how medical decisions and treatments are rendered. Technology is playing a significant role in the vital fields of medicine and targets the services of smart healthcare in three different sectors: clinical institutions, regional health institutes, and individual family members. These entities are interconnected through applications that consist of virtual assistance, smart health centers, patient diagnosis, and patient treatment. Deloitte indicated that technologies such as nanotechnology, genomics, blockchain, augmented reality (AR), additive manufacturing, robotics, and cognitive computing made medical care less expensive and more versatile for caretakers and patients. The report also indicated that new devices (both handheld and wearable) make it possible to collect the patients' data remotely in an efficient way [3].

The evolution of these technologies has opened new opportunities and possibilities in the field of healthcare. Armando observed the adoption of smart healthcare monitoring devices in India and pointed out that the cost varies according to the features and design of the device. Despite this it is investigated how these devices can have a remarkable effect in developing countries that have reduced treatment cost and patient time at the same level [5].

The rising trend of remote healthcare allows for a timelier administration of treatment for patients at their homes, significantly reducing the cost of intervention as well as improving the quality of care with personalized technologies. The patients can decide whether or not to further consult healthcare professionals. The automated computational readings of smart devices refer consultation of a physician to seek emotional support and inpatient care. For personalized care, patients may also use applications to detect a correspondence between the condition and medication interactions to make the decisions on how to improve their health. Furthermore, for more in-depth testing, patients may also decide to use home kits or personalized genomic services. Smart healthcare technology consists of different components such as sensors, smart pills, smart surgeries, wearables, and registration devices. Remote technologies may help healthcare professionals to provide fast and better care.

Technologies such as cloud computing, artificial intelligence (AI), 3D printing, Internet of Things (IoT), 5G, and blockchain revolutionized our physical world by doing a digital replacement of real-world objects with virtual ones. In this chapter, we discuss the role of emergent technologies (such as AI and blockchain), their usage, and applications in smart healthcare. AI is leveraged to make predictions based on the learned patterns and experience of the machines. 5G is another emerging technology, which is currently in its commercialization phase. Similarly, blockchain, a distributed ledger, is used for data and transaction transparency as well as immutability. Once the data has been recorded in the blockchain, it becomes immutable. Shou [1] indicated that the problems of existing smart healthcare are not only dependent on technological advancement but also a joint venture of doctors, patients, and health institutions related to cost reduction, management of diagnostics and data, which improves patients' feedback. Yin et al. [6] discuss implantable and wearable medical devices that gather physical signals from anywhere and anytime, which are based on IoT and machine learning. The world is facing numerous health crises in case of surgeries, treatments, and ever-increasing demands of medicines, but all of these crises will be tackled by the emergence of smart care technologies in the health sector.

1.2 Emerging Technologies in Smart Healthcare

Several technologies are revolutionizing the field of healthcare, from the process of diagnosis until final treatment. At this stage, the role of technology is becoming prominent. The Working Party on Biotechnology, Nanotechnology, and Converging Technologies (BNCT) recommends policies for managing emerging technologies for health innovation, converging technologies, and norms of good governance of healthcare [9]. To get healthy it is necessary to receive better results, and there should be an association between patient and doctor for healthier treatments. Treating patients is itself a task, and this task would be done properly by a quality collaboration of patients and healthcare professionals. Misha described a methodological review over the healthcare transformation that showed how computational methods and simulation made a base for evolution in healthcare by facilitating physiological measurement to detect organic systems [7]. Information technology is a world-class example in this field together with biomedical equipment to establish the keystone of smart healthcare.

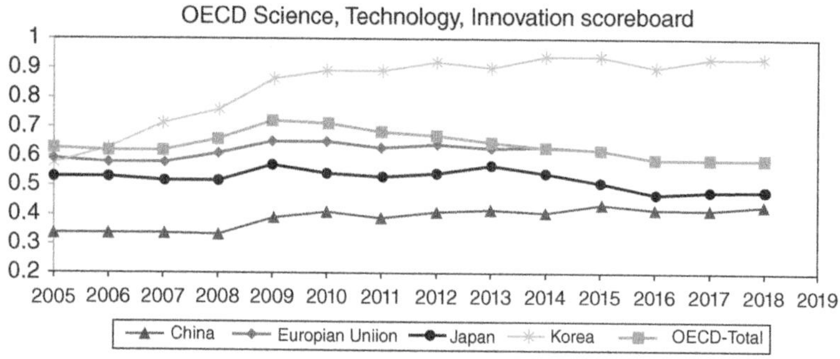

Figure 1.1 OECD countries, science and technology.

OECD (Organisation for Economic Co-operation and Development) countries Science and Technology Scoreboard [8].

Figure 1.1 is a science, technology, and innovation scoreboard in the field of research and development with continuous evolution and enhances data visualization tools. The graph is derived from the OECD (Organisation for Economic Co-operation and Development) database, indicates technological advancement from 2005 to 2019 in China, the European Union, Japan, Korea, and OECD countries, and it indicates Korea became more diverse from 2005 to 2019. The scoreboard contained the indicator of gross domestic expenditure on research and development as a percentage of GDP (Gross Domestic Product) for the countries mentioned in the graph.

1.2.1 Artificial Intelligence (AI) in Healthcare

AI holds great sovereignty in the field of computer technology and is spreading its autonomy among many sectors of the world. One of the main sectors influenced by AI is healthcare as it digitizes human life at a vast level from the life of a single individual to several people's lives. AI is having a great impact on economical, societal, and industrial domains through healthcare and medicine. Some of the roles we define in this chapter such as AI can anticipate the current heart rate of an individual using big data machine learning and expert systems. Another benefit anticipated is that it has made medical care less costly and more available. AI has made it simple for doctors, nurses, and hospital staff to do complex jobs in a very short time and in an efficient manner.

Going through the important medical questions, AI techniques can compile healthcare information from big data sources, which helps in proper decision-making converting these several pen-and-paper-based processes into a digitized form to make computer software more intelligent and autonomous. AI and machine learning are accelerating the cadence of healthcare very quickly. AI aims to recast the medical industry and bring about certain strategies that were unattainable in real scenarios. AI helps analyze and identify patterns in ambiguous datasets more quickly and efficiently. On the other hand, machine learning makes use of learning algorithms to extract attributes from the incoming data (input data is the patients' attributes such as gender, medical history, genetic expression, age, analytical imaging, and symptoms). The OECD AI Principles are the first such principles signed up to by governments. Beyond OECD members, other countries including Argentina, Brazil, Costa Rica, Malta, Peru, Romania, and Ukraine have already adhered to the AI Principles, with further adherents welcomed.

The role of AI is to make computers more beneficial in overcoming healthcare challenges. Various chronic diseases such as diabetes, Alzheimer's, several types of cancers including colon and breast cancer, and cardiovascular diseases are diagnosed early just due to AI.

The recommendation indicates five complementary values-based principles for the responsible management of trustworthy AI:

- AI increases inclusive growth, sustainable development, and well-being.
- AI systems are configured in a way that allows them to act as appropriate safeguards—for example, enabling human intervention where necessary—to ensure smart home gadgets for better living.
- There should be responsible disclosure around AI systems to ensure that people understand AI-based outcomes and can challenge them.
- AI systems must function in a robust, secure, and safe way throughout their life cycles, and potential risks should be continually assessed and managed.
- Organizations and individuals developing, deploying, or operating AI systems should be held accountable for their proper functioning in line with the above principles [12]. We could not imagine our world now without AI.

1.2.2 Internet of Things (IoT) in Smart Healthcare

The term "Things" in IoT in healthcare refers to the network of physical healthcare objects, meaning digital emergent technologies that connect the offline world through the Internet following some standard rules. Healthcare services are interconnected via smart sensors and devices. IoT has been conceived as one of the best solutions to face healthcare challenges and has therefore grabbed the attention of present research. It is supporting remote health monitoring making doctors capable of seeing their patients remotely and supervise them accordingly. IoT is using wireless sensor networks to communicate with doctors and outdoor patients for monitoring. Patients are having several smart types of equipment such as blood glucose monitors, pulse oximeters, blood pressure monitors, pedometers, and weighing scales [17]. With the help of these sensors, patients' important data such as health history, biometric data, treatment history, patient reports, symptoms, and outcome measures that is needed to predict the fitness and future medical care is shared with the doctors. Therefore, it is providing great opportunities to utilize and adopt different monitoring methods for patient caretakers and medical staff. Its benefits cannot be neglected, as remote healthcare is beneficial for critical and noncritical patients as well. It has reduced the burden on hospitals from preventing day-by-day increase cases. IoT has also played a significant role in providing healthcare to patients living in rural areas that don't have adequate access to it. For elder people who are at their homes for a longer period and are unable to make checkups, IoT has also emerged as a convenient resource for them. IoT systems are becoming expedient contributors in the healthcare industry [Impaired patients can be assisted by medical professionals without any waste of time by electronic communication by pointing toward various letters on their device and personal computers so they can call or even ask easily.

A famous term used in describing healthcare services provided through the IoT is "**Telerehabilitation**" and corresponds to the less expensive but the finest service. Regardless of any geographical barriers, it is the best solution for those patients who physically cannot attend the clinics and hospitals. It is most beneficial for older people because of its workability and cost effectiveness for managing their lifestyle and daily routine for doing therapy at home. A survey suggests that primary healthcare costs can be reduced up to 80 percent through telemedicine; this is one of the goals of WHO [18].

In the context of remote monitoring, smart devices allow us to change any rehabilitation tool in IoT devices. Parameters of human health such as body mass, body fat, or mass index can be measured by those devices connected to remote computers via Bluetooth by utilizing bioelectric impedance analysis (BIA) and carrying out periodic analyses of collected data. IoT is also playing a crucial role in cloud-based intelligent healthcare services that keep a real-time check on chronic diseases such as cancer. Health-related data is stored in cloud repositories for future use. The newly emerged infrastructure of cloud computing can be accessed by anyone and anywhere at any time. It has empowered medical professionals to provide the best analysis and assistance for the treatment of disease. It uses principal component analysis (PCA) for characteristic evaluation and the KNN algorithm to monitor patients' health statistics. KNN has a good performance to identify specific diseases, a most valuable and universally accessible healthcare service provided by IoT.

1.2.3 Blockchain in Smart Healthcare

Blockchain is like a powerful synergist to secure healthcare records by providing data integrity and alleviating many challenges in the health sector realm. By attaining, analyzing, and transferring medical information at different levels, blockchain is introduced by researchers to improve the medical field and even aid researchers to unlock genetic codes. Better care, early response of care takers, and timely medicines would be possible if the healthcare system shifted toward electronic and smart gadgets. Effective e-health systems with quick response contain super-quality services and privacy for patients. Blockchain makes us able to interact within untrusted circumstances while keeping privacy and security and enabling a reduced cost [19]. To manage electronic records of patients, blockchain has uncountable opportunities. The traditional system is more rapidly catching the advanced technology, making it more convenient and easier to use for doctors and patients both to maintain the privacy and uprightness of the healthcare system using a blockchain framework named Smart Healthcare System (SHS). Due to its transparency, blockchain has extended to many healthcare domains. Data in the form of blocks is related via cryptographic methods and a decentralized database is then shared between all the peers so that anyone can view and access it. Each block is having its unique ID. These IDs, or hashes, are being generated for every incoming block containing new content, and each block carries the hash of every block that follows (hence the name blockchain). Blockchain is also beneficial for the insurance companies and pharmaceutical industry by keeping their records secure and safe. The data once kept in the block remains part of it for further research and diagnosis and make it possible to track the availability of medicines and medical equipment [20].

1.2.4 3-Dimensional (3D) in Smart Healthcare

3D printing is a manufacturing technology that can physically design a model by fusing or decomposing materials such as resin, plastics, metal, carbon fiber, nitinol, paper, graphite, powder, and many different products. This method is also referred to as additive manufacturing (AM), rapid prototyping, or solid freeform fabrication. It can produce an object of any shape and size as visualize by a computer drawing file. It constructs the object layer by layer by injecting the material with the help of a printhead, a nozzle, or other various printing technologies. It first builds the basic object model along an x-y plane and then subsequently starts building it along the z-axis vertically. These instructions are being followed by a CAD file. 3D printers adopt the step-by-step instructions and deposit the material layer by layer, which results in a real-time object model, and this model is being equipped with scaling, mudding, or painting if required.

Due to life-changing innovations in 3D printing, most industries have started adopting its techniques because of its wonderful results. The healthcare industry has also been greatly affected by 3D printing because its emergence has overcome some challenges that not long ago seemed unsurmountable. Let us discuss some revolutionary changes that 3D printing has enabled in the healthcare sector. According to a survey, almost 6 percent of healthcare professionals have adopted this technology while the rest of them are in the process of adopting it. The most appealing 3D printing laboratory was found in New South Wales, and several skilled workers were hired to provide the services in the lab. They provide patients with such operational products that helps them to fulfill difficult tasks. The surgical tools and devices printed can help patients to improve their anatomy.

3D printing technologies that have been used in healthcare include orthotics prosthetics, implants, and preoperational models. 3D printing design models have specific customers whom they help to perform their activities in a better way. It can reduce patient visits to a hospital and can build such a difficult model that cannot be obtained by any other method. It uses materials such as polypropylene whose mechanical properties make the final product light in weight and easy to hold for patients.

1.2.5 Fifth Generation (5G) in Smart Healthcare

The emerging technologies discussed before having contributed a great part in smart medication, telemedicine, and to provide remote assistance to the patients. Another smart technology named 5G is currently one of the fastest growing industries. 5G is proposed by researchers and experts to continue to assist and monitor patients in several diseases. Smartly designed gadgets and sensors collect information from a number of resources and provide guidance to anyone from anywhere to assist them in taking the right medication in the right manner so that the mistakes can be prevented to use medicines as well as to reduce the cost of treatments and medicines [21].

5G is the upcoming generation of today's 4G network, so 5G can deliver the speedy, extensible network having the larger volume. Instead of providing the fastest Internet connection, the healthcare industry is also getting benefit due to 5G's reliable connectivity for heavy medical devices with increased spectrum, greater capacity, more users as compared to previous LTE networks. 5G can technically provide a low latency of 1 ms, as compared to the previous 20 ms latency. It is good enough to strengthen medical sensors and devices, medical equipment, and video streaming, which may be helpful in telemedicine, teleconsultation, and remote surgery with clean streaming and detailed information deliverance. 5G has also overcome the data transfer issues faced in high-latency networks with stable high speed. 5G provides a greater number of facilities as compared to 4G in smart diabetes detection. It can provide the following **five benefits** to the patients as well as paramedical staff.

- **Profitability:** It makes users aware of a pre-diabetic condition if there is one and provides them with a healthy way of life, which can save their expenditures on treatment and medicines For older people who are long-term patients and unable to attend doctors, it provides tele-treatment.
- **Convenience:** 5G does not discomfort the patient as it supports smart-clothing glucose monitoring. Another instance is that healthcare providers are extending their duties outside the hospital through real-time video conferencing.
- **Personification:** 5G uses several machine learning algorithms and different computing techniques for the prevention of diabetes. Depending on patients' health records, 5G generates a personalized treatment for e patient.
- **Durability:** 5G supports efficient sharing of useful information between doctors and patients and friends and family to change the mental condition of patients so that they can feel self-motivated and produce good changes in their environment and be prepared for a better future treatment.
- **Elegance:** With its intellectual characteristics toward patient health and resources, it can detect diabetes sooner and prevent its causes.

1.3 Realization of SHC through Emerging Technologies (Applications)

1.3.1 Applications of AI

Early detection of healthcare conditions, smart diagnosis, telemedicine, and discovery of several treatments are possible due to the emergence of AI. AI in healthcare produces an advantage in care and quality services. Smart healthcare is a supreme platform for AI applications and systems, where the health industry depends on information and logic to improve the patient's state. There has been a fantastic improvement in the collection of data containing genetic, environmental, mental, and behavioral information. If we use AI in our daily healthcare routine, then it will not only improve our health condition, but it will also recognize the detection and upcoming illness occurring in our body. Some of the important facts of health where AI goes revolutionize this sector with its full zoom. Fei Jiang illustrates the analytical techniques of AI in healthcare either structured in modern deep learning and neural networks or unstructured in terms of natural language processing (NLP). AI uses algorithms to take structures from the bulk of healthcare data and target them to assist in the clinic. This paper mentions the future of AI and surveys its application for managing the healthcare system [4].

1.3.1.1 Patient Care Improvement

Patient care in terms of clinical and in home-based settings have both been greatly enhanced by AI. In the healthcare sector AI plays the role of a backbone for developing and improving patient care in predictive analytics and decision support systems. OECD hosted a Global Partnership on AI (GPAI) that directs the route of AI to behave responsibly in respecting patients' rights by bridging the gap between experts from academia, civilians, stakeholders, and industry by proper implementation of theory and practice [13, 14]. Precision medicine can take part in improving patient health by recruiting complex datasets from a variety of complex situations, for example, health records, morphological data, and psychological reactions. AI-enhanced technologies can point out dangerous conditions or encourage emotional health. These technologies are more beneficial for older people and people having special abnormalities.

1.3.1.2 Maintaining Health Records

Medical practice has become transformed due to computerized patient healthcare charts. Electronic health record (EHR) systems are increasingly adopted in many developed countries; they also establish mobile health to allow mobile services in support with the usage of medicines for daily health routine checkups. EHR systems diminish errors of medication and improve coordination of care. The data extracted from EHR systems for statistics and research give support to many countries to achieve the goal for a high-level achievement. Healthcare still captures the data in devices and is separately analyzed. Interoperability is a basic challenge that must be known about the full future of EHRs. One of the articles described the situation of young man, Roger, who came to the hospital in emergency grumbling with nausea and belly pain. This article showed 55 doctors to identify the usability of EHRs. These digital versions of paper charts are used by caretakers to record patients' history, lab tests, early diagnosed prescriptions, disease background, and so forth, for medication doctor transfer in the EHR system and the search contained 500-mg dosage of Tylenol because Roger was 26 years old. The doctor selected the appropriate option and prescribed the medication dose [16]. Availability of data is a basic element of EHR implementation, and EHR makes a perfect match for machine learning for fueling the data science operations. Machine learning is a remarkable milestone for fundamentals of EHR for example, data mining, NLP for document searching, transcription of report generation, data visualization, privatization and data, and predictive analysis. Thus we can say without AI we cannot imagine the medical world today.

1.3.2 Applications of IoT

IoT made the profession of healthcare more vigilantly connected with a survivor. Chronic diseases are increasing very fast and the population is aging, so there is a deep necessity of connectivity with pocket devices that can be easily accessible for both patients and doctors. Most people have a scarce situation to fight with the basics of healthcare but emerging technology at least IoT can ensure access to healthcare accessories easily and help to reach your doorstep. IoT has a significant role in healthcare innovations; according to statistical projections the use of healthcare devices is anticipated to increase to about 25.8 million units by 2025 [18]. From many types of research, IoT for healthcare in the context of remote patient monitoring for the care of the patient through sensor usage by gathering and inspecting the data and sending inspected patients' information remote to the hospitals and care organization allows for prescribed quick action [11]. Sensors, digital assistance, and radio frequency identification tags (RFID) are made pervasive to collect on-time data and help to make quick decisions. Controlling and monitoring play an important role for the implementation of IoT [10].

1.3.2.1 Glucose Monitoring

Diabetes is now becoming a common disease in developing countries due to unhealthy environments and food processing; older people is especially affected so they must watch their glucose levels to avoid any bad situation. IoT introduces a glucose monitoring system for continuous surveillance. Diabetes patients would have devices equipped with sensors embedded below their dermis. The sensor in the device sends continuous signals toward the personal gadget when glucose level is too low and stores history for them too. In this way, the patient will intelligently know when the circumstances are at risk due to the shortage of glucose in the present scenario as well as in the future.

1.3.2.2 Monitoring Heart Rate

Devices can detect the heart rates; these devices are used by patients. High blood pressure would be diagnosed by this wearable device. The heart rate is continuously recorded by the patient's device that can be sensed with the connection of a patient's body. Healthcare providers will have an approach to monitoring the patient's heart rate whenever they will need to do a check-up. The examined heart rate provided the data, which will be useful for further treatment and diagnosis. In the same way, the wearable devices can notify the health care professionals when the patient suffers strokes, arrhythmias, and heart attacks. In this dangerous situation, the healthcare staff will be on full alert and will be able to dispatch the ambulances in a very timely manner, which can save a patient's life.

1.3.2.3 Smart Inhalers

These IoT inhalers are intelligent with advanced digital features, linked with an application in a smartphone or some gadget that transmits information about what patients need to do to handle this condition. When a patient is experiencing an asthma attack, the transmitted instructions are sent toward the caregivers for them to provide care on time. Some of the inhalers contain sensors that can sense the polluted environment and regions that have high pollen; the sensors help to send a message for the reminder to check the technology of inhaler. They all are equipped smartly to trace how often an inhaler is to be used so the patient does not require to keep records. One of the main facts about these smart inhalers is that they remind victims when to take their medication.

1.3.3 Application of Blockchain

Blockchain has a broad extent of applications and usages in the field of healthcare. The secure relocation of patients' information keeps health records and management of medical grant chains, all of them due to facilitation of ledger technology. It also helps the researchers to unlatch genetic code. In September 2015, a World Economic Forum report was delivered, which surveyed that 58 percent of respondents said 10 percent of all globe domestic products will be stocked by blockchain technology by the year 2025 [19]. Nichol described Healthbank, Swedish based on health system transactions in the blockchain. Their aim is to introduce a unique way of sharing data and securing personal data. For future endeavors the patient health information (for example, blood pressure, heartbeat rate, eating habits, and sleeping pattern) would be fetched from healthcare applications, career appointments all of which be safely stored in the health bank blockchain [15].

1.3.3.1 Stability of Patients' Data

In healthcare, nowadays the foremost data of healthcare is used for retaining the security and safety, which is considered as the eminent application of blockchain. Keeping data sealed is a valuable issue in the health sector. Blockchain presents a stable, secure, decentralized, and transparent log of patients' data and becomes a widespread security application in this field. From complex and secure code it can conceal the user's identity privately from massive codes that enable the maturity of sensitivity. The decentralized nature of blockchain presents the same information to doctors, nurses, paramedic staff, and also patients quickly and securely. Mettler described one of the Netherland-based security organization partners with the Estonia government, who implemented Guardtime, to facilitate the framework of blockchain to authenticate the patients' identity [21].

1.3.3.2 Distant Patient Monitoring

Distant patient monitoring is itself a technology that authorizes the status of the patient outside of traditional clinic systems e.g. In separate regions or homes which may need to increase the patient's care and reduce the phenomenal cost. In this case, blockchain plays a vital role for monitoring. In distant patients monitoring the caregiver staff would be able to know the status of the patient, the medical record is collected through smart devices and IoT networks. For cache, allotment, and rectify the medical information Blockchain playing an important role in all of these tasks. Ray described the connectivity of IoT with blockchain for retrieving, sharing, and storing electronic health information in the form of data flow architecture [21]. Distant patient monitoring becomes valuable for the elderly patient and disabled patients because they can take quick steps to save their lives. Many kinds of research show that blockchain is the key factor to save the patient data securely and manageable, in this context Ichikawa illustrated cognitive therapy for the disease of insomnia for patients monitoring by adopting a hyper ledger fabric architecture.

1.3.3.3 Blockchain Prevents Costly Mistakes

Blockchain can provide a single platform for saving and continuously updating health records for private and on-time retrieval by authorized users. By circumventing miscommunication among several healthcare professionals contained in the knowledge of patients, prevented by many mistakes, faster diagnosis and mediation become possible, as well as personalized care for every patient. Medical professionals cost the healthcare sector whenever miscommunication has occurred. The time taken to access the patients' data irritates caretakers and delays in the care of the patient. Blockchain dispenses a cure for all this time taken and costly errors.

1.3.4 Applications of 3D Printing

3D printing is used to create new cells and tissues for active regenerative processes. 3D printing is a relatively expanded, unique, smart method of producing that established various applications in defense, aerospace, dentistry, organs fabrication, and in many other areas. In this section we discuss the revolutionary effect of 3D bioprinting in healthcare. Assistance obtained by application of 3D printing in medicine does not only include personalized medical products and equipment but also high productivity, cost effectiveness, design moralization, and increased collaboration. The application of 3D printing is going to be mainstream.

1.3.4.1 Hearing Aids

In this sphere, the efforts were originated by Belgium-based organization Materialize [22], in collaboration with production of Swiss hearing aids. Phil Reeves discusses the 3D printing revolution; more than 10 000 000 3D printed hearing assistance devices are currently used worldwide. There are many more that are in use today. Nowadays 3D printing, which includes scanning, modeling, and printing, takes less than a day.

1.3.4.2 3D Printing in Rejuvenate Medicine and Fight with Covid-19 Pandemic

In this neoteric era the creation of tissues from fluffy biomaterial such as biomimetic polymers and living cells has been the most remarkable technological advancement in this field. Since the early 2000s, simple organs such as the bladder have been embedded into the patient. Moreover, various difficulties need to be resolved for intricate organs such as the liver, heart, and brain to be 3D-printed and then placed into a patient's body. The rapid action of Covid-19 has placed great stress on medical systems all over the world, with stipulation of censorious medical kits and equipment. Manufacturers have responded to supply medical gadgets for hospitals. Carbon and 3D systems have started to be used for manufacturing open-source PPE for health staff workers worldwide.

1.4 Conclusion

In this chapter, the deployment of the framework for healthcare in IoT distinguishes the applications from the physical infrastructure; therefore, we suggest to develop the platform for healthcare with the different emerging technologies. We have thereby discussed the technologies benefitting and challenges on how IoT, 3D printing, AI, and blockchain can help healthcare organizations to enhance the reliability and accessibility of services and various benefits and challenges faced so that Wi-Fi networks are widely used in the healthcare industry.

Author Biography

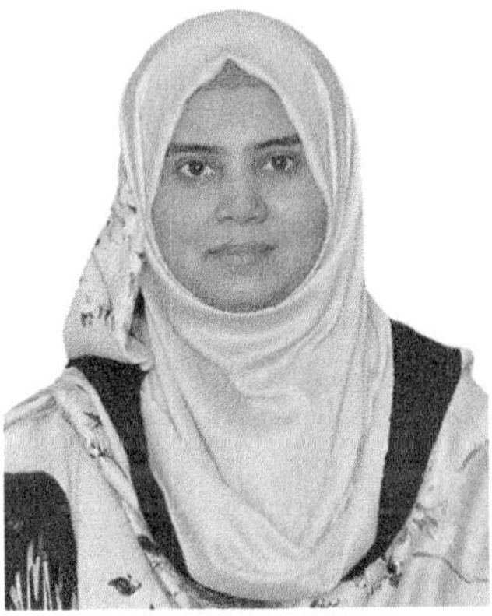

Masooma Zehra Syeda, received her master's degree in Human Computer Interaction & Robotics from Korea Institute of Science and Technology, South Korea in 2017. She has been worked for Indus university Karachi. Her Current research interest includes Human Computer Interaction, Artificial Intelligence, social content services, User interface, Tangible media technology and web content technology.

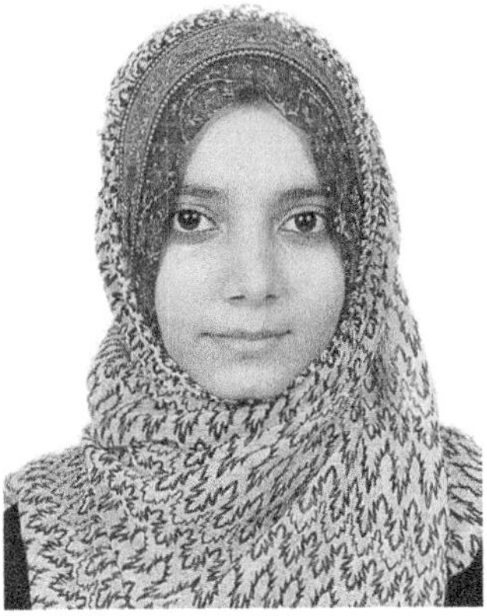

Dur-e-hassan Syeda currently pursuing the bachelor's degree in Software Engineering from Mehran University of Science and Technology Pakistan. Her current research includes Artificial intelligence, machine learning and emotion intelligence.

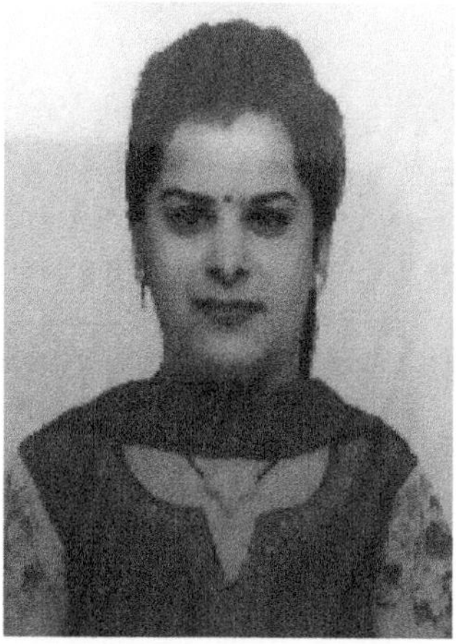

Himanshi Babbar is Assistant Professor-Research in Computer Applications, working in Chitkara University, Rajpura, Punjab, India. She has 2 years of teaching experience, CGC, Landran, Mohali, Punjab. She had Completed MCA (Master's in Computer Applications) from Chitkara University, Punjab Campus and currently Pursuing a Ph.D. in Computer Applications from Chitkara University, Punjab Campus. Her area of research is Software Defined Networking, Load Balancing and Internet of Things. She has attended six national conferences, published many papers in National and International Journals and filed 8 patents.

References

1 Tian, S., Yang, W., Grange, J. et al. (2019). Smart healthcare: making medical care more intelligent. *Global Health Journal* 3: 62–65.

2 Jonathan Skinner, Geisel School of Medicine and Department of Economics, Dartmouth and Amitabh Chandra, Harvard Kennedy School of Government, Harvard Last update: 3 January 2018, Managing new health technologies. https://www.oecd-ilibrary.org/sites/fe499baf-en/index.html?itemId=/content/paper/fe499baf-en.

3 OECD Home, Directorate for Science, Technology and Innovation. https://www.oecd.org/sti/emerging-tech 10-12-2020

4 Fei Jiang, Yong Jiang, Hui Zhi, Yi Dong, Hao Li, Sufeng Ma, Yilong Wang, Qiang Dong, Haipeng Shen, Yongjun Wang, Artificial intelligence in healthcare: past, present and future

5 Going digital: making the transformation work for growth and well being, Artificial intelligence, OECD Principles on AI. https://www.oecd.org/going-digital/ai/, launched in 02-2020.

6 Hongxu, Y., Akmandor, O., Mosenia, A., and Jhad, N.K. (2018). Smart Healthcare. *Journal: Foundations and Trends in Electronic Design Automation*, 12: 401–466.

7 ARTIFICIAL INTELLIGENCE: Launch of the Global Partnership on AI. An international coalition for responsible AI that respects human rights and democratic values

8 OECD Science, Technology and Innovation Scoreboard. https://www.oecd.org/innovation/scoreboard.htm, last updated 5-08-2020.

9 Article on AI, Can I Fix Medical Records? https://www.nature.com/articles/d41586-019-03848-y last updated 18-dec-2019

10 Ashton, K. (2009), I could be wrong, but I'm fairly sure the phrase 'Internet of Things' started life as the title of a presentation I made at Procter & Gamble (P&G) in 1999, RFID Journal.

11 How IoT is Boosting Healthcare Application Development, Emorphis Technologies, 11-06-2019.

12 World Economic Forum (2015, September). Deep Shift. Technology Tipping Points and Societal Impact, [Online]. Available: http://www3.weforum.org/docs/WEF_GAC15_Technological_Tipping_ Points_report_2015.pdf.

13 Mettler M. (2016). Blockchain technology in healthcare: the revolution starts here. IEEE 18th International Conference on e-Health Networking, September 14–16, 2016. Piscataway, NJ: IEEE. http://ieeexplore.ieee.org/stamp/stamp.jsp?arnumber=7749510. Accessed March 3, 2017

14 Ray, P.P., Dash, D., Salah, K., and Kumar, N. (2020). Blockchain for IoT-based healthcare: background, consensus, platforms, and use cases. *IEEE Systems Journal* 15: 85–94.

15 P. B. Nichol (2016). Blockchain applications for healthcare, [Online]. Available: http://www.cio.com/article/3042603/innovation/blockchain-applications-for-healthcare.html.

16 Ichikawa, D., Kashiyama, M., and Ueno, T. (2017). Tamper-resistant mobile health using blockchain technology. *JMIR mHealth and uHealth* 5 (7): e111.

17 Gupta, P., Agrawal, D., Chhabra, J., and Dhir, P.K. (2016). IoT based smart healthcare kit. In: *2016 International Conference on Computational Techniques in Information and Communication Technologies (ICCTICT)*, 237–242.

18 Baker, S.B., Xiang, W., and Atkinson, I. (2017). Internet of things for smart healthcare: technologies, challenges, and opportunities. *IEEE Access* 5: 26521–26544.

19 Mettler, M. (2016). Blockchain technology in healthcare: the revolution starts here. In: *2016 IEEE 18th International Conference on e-Health Networking, Applications and Services (Healthcom), IEEE*. 1–3.

20 Tariq, N., Qamar, A., Asim, M., and Khan, F.A. (2020). Blockchain and smart healthcare security: a survey. *Procedia Computer Science* 175: 615–620.

21 Ahad, A., Tahir, M., and Yau, K.L.A. (2019). 5G-based smart healthcare network: architecture, taxonomy, challenges and future research directions. *IEEE Access* 7: 100747–100762.

22 3D printing software services. https://www.materialise.com/, last accessed: 19-08-2021.

2

ICN-Fog Computing for IoT-Based Healthcare: Architecture and Challenges

Divya Gupta[1], Shalli Rani[1], and Syed Hassan Ahmed Shah[2]

[1] *Chitkara University Institute of Engineering and Technology, Chitkara university, Punjab, India*
[2] *Product Specialist, JMA Wireless, USA*

2.1 Introduction

Internet of Things (IoT) is a promising solution toward integration of various technologies and communication solutions. It describes the arranged set of physical objects with improved sensing, detecting, communication, and networking features. Wireless sensor networks (WSNs) is a leading innovation within IoT that refers to the set of spatially dispersed self-sufficient sensors able to monitor and record the environmental factors. WSNs integrate a set of sensor nodes into one network where all the collected information is sent to a central node, i.e., a sink, via wireless communication. The sensor nodes in a WSN may vary from a few to hundreds or even to several thousands; each node is low cost, portable, and easy to deploy. The integration of WSNs with the IoT has huge potential outcomes in the field of healthcare [1]. The networks with intelligent sensing capabilities can help patients and their guardians by providing continuous monitoring, memory upgrade, access to patient medical history, control of health gadgets (HG), and emergency consultation [2, 3]. The IoT is heading toward a revolution, and it will rebuild the medical services area to support social advantages and entrance as well as financial aspects. The ubiquitous computing in healthcare demands continuous monitoring and management of all the individual entities such as persons, medicines, and appliances. The IoT's network connectivity provides support for monitoring, storing, and using health data continuously 24/7. Based on the rapid development in the

IoT-Enabled Smart Healthcare Systems, Services and Applications, First Edition.
Edited by Shalli Rani, Maheswar Rajagopal, Neeraj Kumar and Syed Hassan Ahmed Shah.

healthcare sector, in the next few years, the way medical care is presently given will be changed from clinic-focused, first to clinic-home-adjusted in 2020, and afterward eventually to home-focused in 2030 [4]. This fundamental change requires that the way the assembly and overlap of the IoT designs and innovations for smart spaces and medical services areas be more effectively taken care of.

IoT has changed the way for the whole community, and every user is fully comfortable to receive updates and information online. The rapid increase in the use of health gadgets for the entire world population would correspond to approximately 10 billion gadgets interconnected through networks. The request from patients would be granted by the central server, essentially the cloud. The high computation power and in practice unlimited storage capacity offered by cloud computing (CC) has expanded healthcare services to wearable health-based systems. Despite its numerous advantages, CC fails in some sensitive requirements, namely, real-time response delivery in emergency situations. The large ongoing network traffic to the cloud suffers from unacceptable delays and other issues, resulting in a reduced quality of service (QoS). The issues caused because of direct communication between IoT and cloud could be addressed by introducing a fog layer between IoT and the cloud [5]. Fog computing extends the cloud to the network edge in order to support real-time delivery.

This large strength of IoT devices demands future networking to share information and therefore borrows ideas from information-centric networking (ICN)—a promising future architecture for content delivery using content names unlike IP addresses [6]. There are various merits associated with the ICN to overcome the challenges imposed by IoT networks, which include name-based forwarding, in-network caching, scalability, content level security, and receiver-driven communication. The request from patients would be first granted by in-network ICN nodes caching the required data to offer minimal delay, or by the central server, essentially the cloud, in case of content not cached inside ICN nodes. With the mentioned benefits of reduced delay, better bandwidth utilization, and improved QoS, ICN is seen as an add-on to the existing healthcare framework as a fog node.

This chapter presents a ICN-fog-based healthcare system framework capable of providing real- time services with use of in–network caching inside information-centric networking–fog nodes (IFN). Based on the intelligent computations performed by the smart health gateway in differentiating regular and critical requests, the critical data would be processed by the ICN-fog layer whereas regular data would directly be sent to the cloud for further processing and storage.

The rest of chapter is organized as follows: Section 2.2 presents the benefits of incorporating of ICN in IoT. Section 2.3 presents the use of IoT in the healthcare domain. Section 2.4 gives a complete discussion of the role of fog computing in IoT for delay-sensitive situations. Further, on the basis of healthcare application, the incorporation of fog computing in healthcare is demonstrated in Section 2.5. Section 2.6 describes the architecture of healthcare by leveraging both ICN and fog for fast content delivery. The various challenges facing the healthcare sector leveraging ICN-fog architecture are listed in Section 2.7. Finally, Section 2.8 gives the conclusion of this chapter.

2.2 ICN in IoT

The various challenges presented by the traditional host centric-based IoT communication can be easily addressed using ICN—a future Internet network architecture [6, 7]. Unlike IP-based host-centric communication, which primarily focuses on location, ICN considers the network content as the primary entity and therefore is known to be the new networking paradigm for next Internet generation. This implies ICN supports dynamic establishment of channel based on content names irrespective of static establishment of channel by connecting two end points based on IP address in traditional communication. Further, ICN has gained a lot of popularity and interest due to its promising nature of providing simple, reliable, and secure communication. ICN supports a hierarchical naming convention by providing unique, persistent, and location-independent names for every interest and data packets. All such packets with unique hierarchical name are considered as self-authenticated data by entire ICN network nodes. Any consumer in need to access content from the network can easily get it by specifying the content name without providing any information about device location or any IP address. ICN offers a variety of inherent features such as mobility, security, in-network caching, scalability, flexibility, and ease of data exchange. Till date, there are a total of 9 projects that are incorporating ICN as a base theme with their own design [8]. Among all these network architectures only PURSUIT, NDN, and Mobility First are considered as clean slate architectures while all the rest are known as dirty slate. However, most of them share common features such as name-based communication irrespective of IP address and exchange of packets for communication; they also maintain some data structures for managing data flow between producer and consumer. However, NDN is a prevailing architecture among all the existing architectures. In this regard, the next discussion on the packet types and structures used in general for ICN will be in reference to NDN.

2.2.1 ICN Architecture

In this day and age, the Internet design fixates on the network layer. Figure 2.1 presents the common hour-glass architecture [9, 10] of both IP and NDN. The NDN's network layer underpins effectiveness, dependability, scalability, and content security. In customary host-centric norms, communication is traded after a channel is set up between producer and consumer. It does not support any facility in case of loss of connection; rather, it will in general build up a new channel in the network. The NDN architecture presents two new layers: (i) strategy layer, to support state-full forwarding, and (ii) security layer, to support content security. In NDN, information packets are marked with a producer key to give verification just as secure correspondence.

NDN supports recipient-driven communication with two sorts of trade packets: interest packets and data packets [10]. Both packets themselves convey progressive, application-oriented content names.

The information flow in NDN begins with the recipient sending an interest packet. The packet with content name is sent by the in-network nodes in the network until it arrives at the producer or the respective content isn't retrieved. The content provider reacts sending the data packet with the mentioned content in reverse to the recipient. Data packets carry the name and content being marked by the producer key to verify the information. Data packet travels in reverse to the interest packet. Figure 2.2 shows the packets design in NDN.

2.2.2 ICN Data Structures

2.2.2.1 Content Store (CS)

The in-network nodes in ICN that handle both packets for the most part have three fundamental segments, and the Content Store (CS) is one of them [11]. The CS is a finite capacity temporary storage for caching the named content. In ICN, whenever any node gets an interest packet, its first query is in its temporary store, i.e., CS; if a mentioned name is discovered in CS, at that point the interest will be fulfilled. This implies that every node in an ICN network that handles the information packets will store a duplicate of the information in its CS (in-network reserving) to fulfill any future interest for a similar content. To better utilize network resources, ICN utilizes a few systems and trade approaches for stored named content.

2.2.2.2 Pending Interest Table (PIT)

The Pending Interest Table (PIT) maintains the record of content names and interface of all the interest packets that have been sent by a node but have not been fulfilled yet. As referenced beforehand, when any node gets

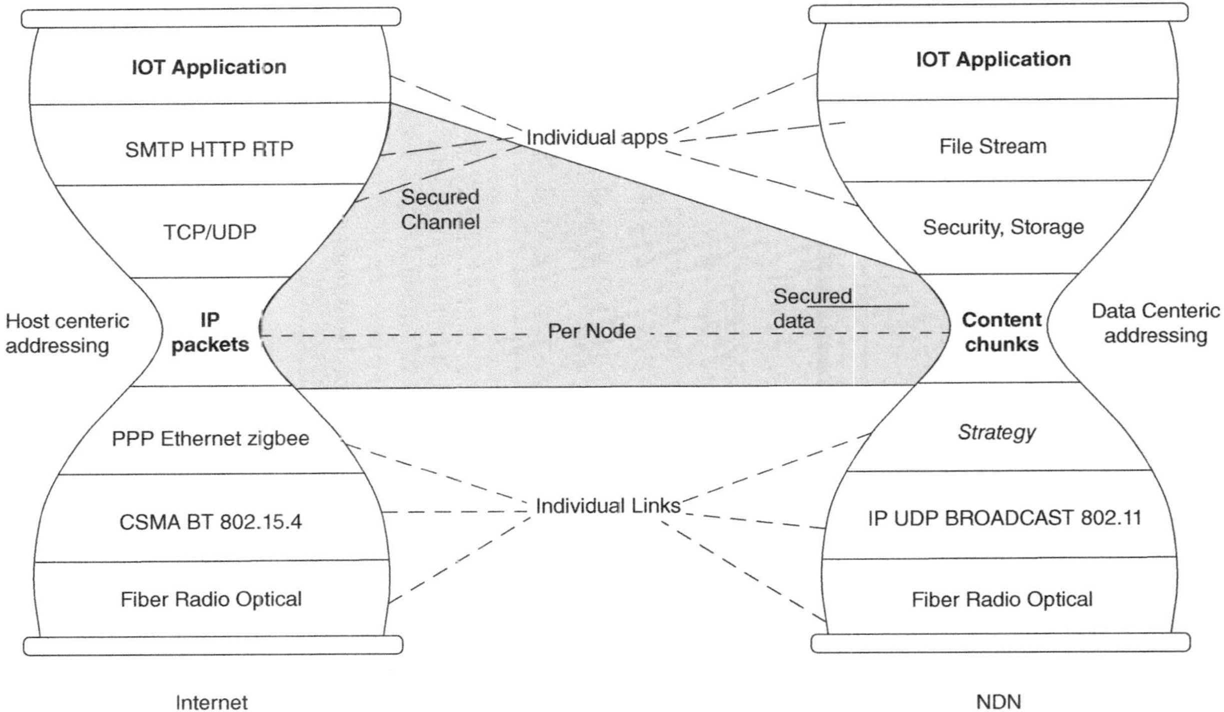

Figure 2.1 NDN hourglass architecture.

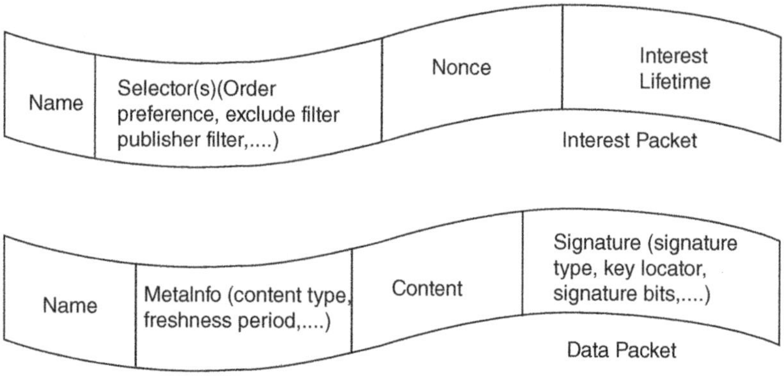

Figure 2.2 NDN packet format.

an interest packet, it initially looks into its CS to fulfill the required information; if the information is not in the CS, the node will make an entry in the PIT comprising the content name in the interest and identifier of the interface from where the interest is received. Afterwards, the interest is sent to the forwarding information base (FIB) for additional preparing. The entry in the PIT will be used later to send the data packet to the reversed path. Data packets with no existing entry in the PIT will be treated as spontaneous and therefore get dropped.

2.2.2.3 Forwarding Information Base (FIB)

The FIB keeps records of outgoing interfaces for incoming interest packets. The packets are forwarded to the next hops based on the longest name prefix matching. Irrespective of IP-based communication, where a single packet is mapped to only one outgoing interface, NDN supports multiple interfaces for a single incoming packet. The selection of a particular interface among the present ones is solely based on forwarding strategies.

2.3 IoT in Healthcare

IoT is changing the medical services and is a widely accepted technology by the general public. Utilizing various sensors to continuously monitor the medical services is one of the most challenging tasks [12]. Limiting the expenses and improving the well-being of the patients and simultaneously managing staff shortages are essential concerns [13]. Figure 2.3 shows the general model representing IoT in healthcare. Healthcare services need multilayer engineering for some specific calculations. With mobile edge

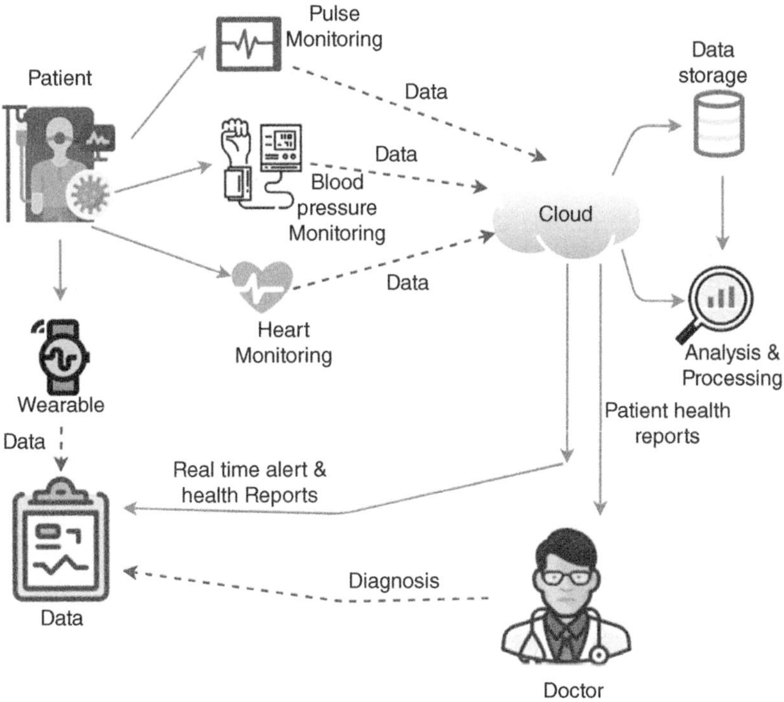

Figure 2.3 IoT in healthcare.

computing, patients' health can be easily monitored even if a patient is located far from the specialist while maintaining a central cloud at a local site. The work in [14] presents a window-based rate control approach (w-RCA) and clinical nature of administration (m-QoS) algorithms, which offer better assistance and quality for mobile edge-based medical care [14]. The real-time collection of patient health data was performed through wearable sensor devices connected to mobile applications. Patients can follow their well-being while at the same time visiting or resting at home whenever and wherever. Farahani et al. [15] state P2P video/sound capabilities can be given to patients to distinguish proof of illnesses in the same way as difference between taking their medicines and to refilling of medication at any required point.

In healthcare, IoT can be particularly valuable especially for older patients. For home care assistance, a self-caution framework was presented by the work in [16] to take the medication. Likewise, the condition of medication bottle is followed by the weight sensors to generate a notice if there is a medication overdose. The works in [17] propose the utilization of radio frequency identification tags (RFID) innovation marks and labels on patients' meds associated over the IoT with the patient's very own clinical records. Utilizing such services, the specialist/doctors can distantly screen the patient well-being, and a notification will be sent to doctors or attendants if certain adjustments are required in the previous state. The work uses AI calculations and a probabilistic learning structure using classification techniques to improve the accuracy. Further, the work in [18], proposes a necklace to track the amount of medicine intake by patients. It works by noticing the neck skin movement while they take the medication.

IoT for ambient assisted living (AAL) is primarily focused toward comfortable and satisfactory life of individuals who are not independent anymore and are staying at home. It not only allows to check patients' health and well-being but also their comfort. The gadgets and items would be associated with one another to help the old, impaired people in their everyday scheduled exercises [19]. It will likewise deal with the development of illnesses by real-time monitoring of patients' fundamental indicators. IoT in healthcare provides new hopes for patients as well as old individuals; however, the consistent association among areas, patients, and emergency clinics isn't really easy to accomplish. The primary challenges for IoT in healthcare mainly comprises: (i) The management of huge amounts of data collected through different sensors attached to a single patient. In addition to that, data collected in dynamic state with all the movements in a patient's body is more challenging; (ii) The variety of data collected among different patients may require specific handling and analysis. For example, some patients' data may be collected by sensors in the form of images and for some it might be in text format; (iii) IoT in healthcare is always time specific and need real-time processing. More specifically, latency is not at all tolerable for emergency situations as it may endanger patient's lives. Even IoT in healthcare offers a number of benefits, though it has some challenges, which must be addressed to support more reliable, secure real-time services.

2.4 Role of Fog Computing in IoT

The pay-per-use cloud computing models are an effective option in contrast to claiming or purchasing private data centers. Cloud computing offers various advantages, which include better network resource utilization without compromising performance, easy location tracking with low power requirement, and lower OPEX accomplished through similar storage and networking parts [20]. The latter becomes a drawback for extremely critical applications, where immediate response is key. IoT always requires portability support and geo-dispersion along with location information and reduced delay. The new paradigm to offer such services is known as fog computing, or just fog, as it is accessible before the cloud [20, 21].

Fog computing is actually a virtual platform acting as an interface between cloud data centers and end users by providing different computation, storage, and networking services regularly yet not only situated at the edge of the network. Figure 2.4 presents the data computing and processing design supporting the future IoT applications and outlines the role of fog computing. The computation, storage, and networking services come under the core structure units of both cloud and fog computing. However, edge computing infers various qualities that make fog a non-inconsequential augmentation of the cloud, and this majorly includes location awareness, reduced latency, support for mobility, geo-dispersion, real-time analysis, heterogeneity, large-size networks, and online analysis support with the cloud. Fog computing plays a major role in various IoT application areas that include but are not limited to connected vehicles, smart grid, smart

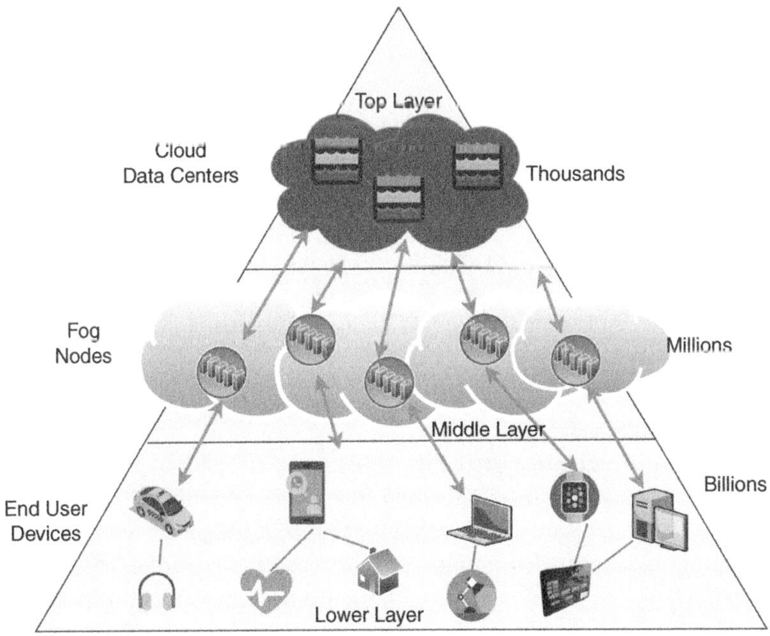

Figure 2.4 Fog computing in IoT.

homes, smart city, healthcare, and WSNs. In this chapter, our focus will be mainly on the use of fog computing for the healthcare domain using ICN network features to support real-time delay-free services.

2.5 Fog Computing in Healthcare: A Classification Approach

Fog computing in healthcare comes with various components to design a real-world solution to the current challenges in this domain. The main components include:

2.5.1 Patient Data

Data about the health of a patient is a significant part of proposed scientific categorization and examined in detail in the following subsections. In recent years, the use of fog computing in the healthcare sector has gained a lot of popularity among different research groups/individuals. There are many works about identification, observation, diagnosis, examination, and representation of sickness when contrasted with previous years. The scientific categorization layout for FC Healthcare is as follows:

2.5.1.1 Data Gathering

The ongoing observation of health and well-being by utilizing wireless body area sensors as well as through several wearable devices has come up as a new developing edge in healthcare. There are rapid advancements in biomedical sensors and remote organization, which accomplished this plan. While discussing persistent monitoring of the human state, the sensing gadgets gather all the necessary data from the patient's body. Further, Vora et al. in [22, 23] examined the qualities and assistance of FC in the healthcare space.

2.5.1.2 Data Examination

In reality, there is a huge gap between the capacity and energy necessities of the long-haul constant observation framework and the proficiencies of existing gadgets/devices. The systems for test aggregation, compressive detecting, and oddity-driven transmission decrease the burden of wireless transmission, compression, information collection, and validation of information. To continuously monitor well-being in real time utilizing worldwide health monitoring systems, the framework ought to have a capacity to acquire bio-signals from sensor gadgets and transmit sensed information to the gateway utilizing particular communication protocols, for example, Wi-Fi. From that point forward, the information is forwarded to distant cloud data centers for preparation, analysis, and representation.

2.5.1.3 Fog Node Organization

A fog node comprises networking gadgets, network conventions, servers, and cloudlets. The demand for sensing devices and the data sensed by these devices is increasing with each passing day leading a constraint regarding node power and communication as well as battery life. To better manage these issues, the work in [24] proposed an FC-based IoT protocol called Message Queue Telemetry Transport (MQTT) by introducing a reduced complexity and computation layer between the cloud and IoT devices. As a rising healthcare float, medical cyber physical systems (MCPSs) enable insightful and close association among the clinical gadgets and computational items. Cloud assets are commonly presented to handle the detected information of clinical gadgets to help MCPSs. On the other hand, long-delay, insecure connections are set up between clinical gadgets and an information focal point of the cloud because of requesting QoS from the MCPS.

2.5.1.4 Health Administrations

The following two components fall into this category.

2.5.1.4.1 Health Gadgets The authors in [24] present a cloud-based healthcare system (CHS), comprising wearable sensors, customized clinical gadgets, transmitters to send the sensed information, and the cloud server for service delivery over the Internet. A clinical cloud has a created application, which speaks with clinical gadgets and furthermore, with sensors sending information from one party to another, for example, patient to doctor. The amendment of the administration has been completed by a specialist ICT framework and a clinical master, in case of getting an alarm for issues during examination of sensed information.

2.5.1.4.2 Applications Among all the cloud-oriented healthcare applications, eHealth attracts extraordinary attention because of its basic prerequisites, and social interest. In healthcare, time is a critical factor in case of emergency. An interference-free crisis-ready framework was tended to by Aazam and Huh [25] called emergency help alert mobile cloud (E-HAMC) framework. This framework utilized the FC for crisis-ready help. E-HAMC is an advanced cell-based help that gives a rapid method for alerting the emergency managing offices.

2.6 ICN-Fog Leveraging Healthcare Architecture

In this section, we describe a three-layer fog-based healthcare architecture using an ICN-IoT gateway that will eventually change the way emergency clinics, centers, and specialists provide healthcare to their patients. The architectural design in Figure 2.5 comprises three principal layers: (i) health gadgets layer (HGL), information-centric networking fog computing layer (IFCL), and cloud layer (CL). It gives a total arrangement from information gathering, information preparing, and enormous information investigation/examination to the cloud stage.

2.6.1 Health Gadgets Layer

An enormous arrangement of IoT-based health gadgets (HG), for example, wearable devices, sensors, and cell phones, comprise the patient-driven medical care framework to monitor the constant well-being and status of patients. The real-time monitoring could be done by any PC or mobile device progressively; the device could coordinate the data securely with the cloud eHealth stage [26]. The design of the healthcare framework leveraging ICN-fog is presented in Figure 2.5. The HGL is the main layer, where various wearables or sensors, for example, a wrist band, smart eyeglasses, and smart watches, are utilized to gather the patient's health information. All they need to have is an association utilizing an appropriate communication protocol through a smart gateway. The legitimate connection establishment could be better achieved by utilizing WSNs or personal area networks (PANs) protocols, for example, Wi-Fi for distant associations and Bluetooth low energy (BLE) for short separation associations. Moreover, the IoT-based health gadgets can be partitioned into two parts: (i) physical brilliant sensors are utilized to carefully screen patients' well-being and track their actual health such as gadgets for monitoring blood pressure, pulse rate, ECG, glucose level, and heartbeat and (ii) virtual brilliant sensors, which are utilized to catch the patients' well-being data and logical information from the remote locations as well as support remote consultations. Such sensors are really easy to operate, cheap, and highly reliable. In this regard, these can be comprehensively conveyed at different public medical clinics or hospitals to screen the patients' well-being and status in real time. These geospatially disseminated sensors produce tremendous detecting information streams, which must be handled cautiously.

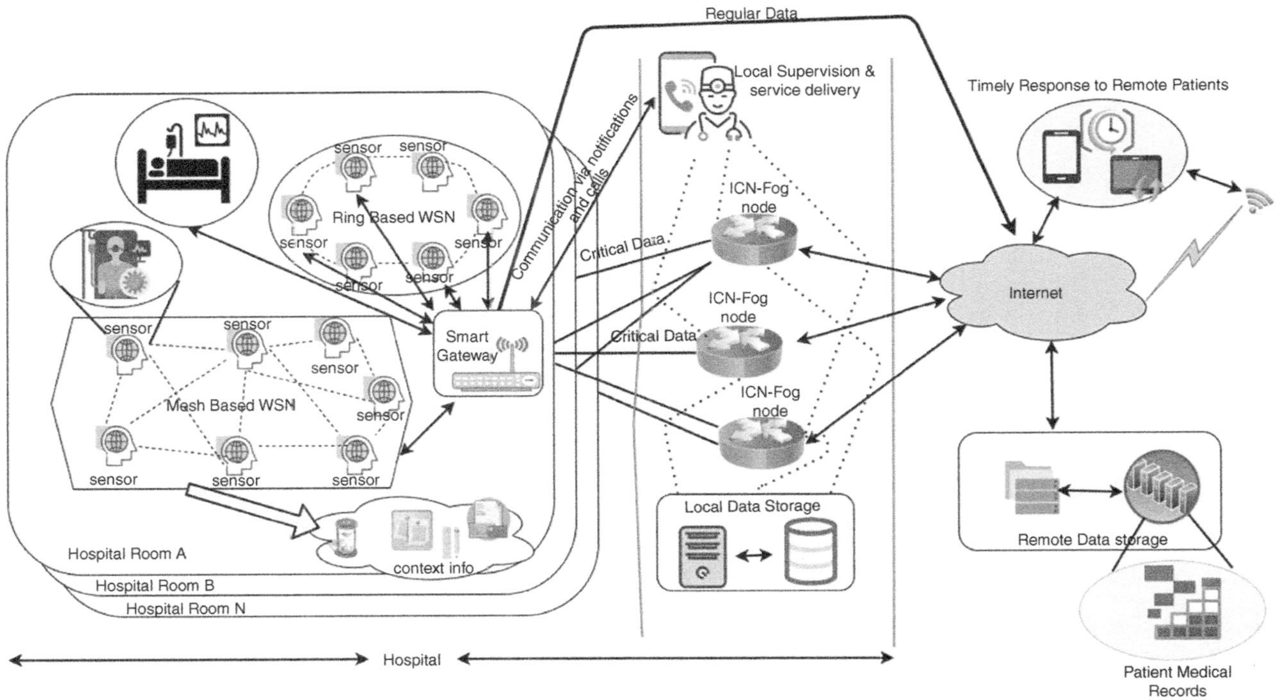

Figure 2.5 ICN-Fog computing in healthcare.

2.6.2 ICN-Fog Computing Layer

The raw data collected from various health gadgets in the first layer, i.e., HGL, is sent to the second layer—IFCL—for further processing and information examination. The IFCL mainly comprises various IFN with low power requirements and high performance gains. Each IFN is associated with a neighborhood gathering of health gadgets that normally covers a little network and perform analysis on data. Real-time computations and low latency are the actual requirements of healthcare systems. IFCL addresses all the difficulties of healthcare by working with CC, big data, ICN, and fog-based frameworks. Without any doubt, it is one of the basic necessities from healthcare to quickly react to time-sensitive information. The traditional cloud computing models to gather and examine the patient's delicate continuous information over a wide geological region is a tedious task and a challenge to implement in healthcare with real-time response requirements. The best strategy to handle these issues is to utilize ICN with fog to continue the CC and its administrations to a different level. The ICN-fog layer handles the difficult piece of the off-path caching. The addition of fog nodes with ICN makes it a suitable candidate for all the patients connected through various health gadgets. The difficulties in allotting IP delivers to all the patient requests and gathered data are accordingly limited by content-driven naming. Further, for resolution of naming conventions, any of the choices—flat, hierarchical, or hash naming—could be preferred. Whereas to make a caching decision, predictive distribution based on publisher-subscriber path will help connect a private cloud to the public cloud. The IFNs are placed near the health gadgets to provide real-time computations for delay-sensitive applications, and rest data could be sent to the cloud for storage. Further, the better network bandwidth utilization could be only achieved by transferring vast amounts of data to FN and then to the cloud after several compressions and filters. Fog computation offers a reliable solution toward reduced latency and high network performance by improved bandwidth utilization.

2.6.3 Cloud Layer

The top-most layer in our healthcare architecture is CL, which comprises high computation data center and a large area monitoring and gives unified control. Due to high computation and large capacity limits of the data center, various complex calculations, relationship modeling, and various pattern recognitions are supportable in this layer. The cloud servers can make dynamic decisions. In addition to that, cloud servers are also responsible for storing the information collected from the fog nodes and some additional information. This information can be given to patients or clinical specialists for charging or outline purposes. Patients can check their current and verifiable clinical history utilizing a portable application or a web interface.

The CL layer itself comprises different inward layers such as:

2.6.3.1 Connection Layer

The responsibility of this layer is to build an association among health gadgets, FNs, and the cloud. FNs and eHealth keen gadgets can be associated with the cloud utilizing any equipment by means of any correspondence channel, for example, 3G/4G, in view of various conventions such as WebSocket.

2.6.3.2 Data Management Layer

This layer incorporates the cloud information from various sources. Further, information is coordinated impeccably with non-sensor sources such as information from e-solution sites, EHRs, and web sources. Thus, knowledgeable clinical specialists can get to the information whenever and whenever is required. It extensively expands the cooperation over all orders expanding the proficiency of healthcare.

2.6.3.3 Application Layer

This layer gives diverse application administrations, for example, enormous information examination, rule motor to make suitable alerts, occasions, notices, and trigger activities.

2.7 Challenges in the Healthcare System

There are several issues and difficulties related with the best possible usage of ICN-fog based healthcare systems. These issues are relevant in terms of services and must be addressed before implementing the healthcare frameworks in the real world:

2.7.1 Organization of Data

The health gadgets acquire a tremendous measure of patients' information, which experiences 5 Vs that correspond to big data: variety, volume, value, veracity, and velocity. This is more identified with the capacities of FN to get, store, measure, and forward. The information variance between fog nodes and the cloud data center needs monitoring from various authoritative arrangements of the framework. Moreover, to deal with the exceptionally divergent information, for example, text, pictures, document, and so on, coming from various sources, for example, a cell phone and a smart watch, standard protocols and information design are needed in FL. Further, the gateway must have proper routing strategies to route routine data as well as critical data.

2.7.2 Usage of Health Gadgets

A major part of the proposed system answers for medical services that comprise wearable gadgets. These gadgets may not be fully protected and there are likewise feelings of unease with these gadgets. Specialists must be prepared and trained to use the IoT; usually they don't know about these advances. It would be too costly to prepare all the clinical staff.

2.7.3 Privacy and Security

The protection of patient data by maintaining privacy and security is a key factor in any healthcare system. If there are accessibility of gadgets, there might happen situations where some patients require all the assets for themselves and deny them to the other patients. This is known as asset hacking in the systems administration area. Utilizing cryptographic methods, privacy can be achieved while exchanging information among clients and machines or workers. In other words, they keep information hidden. To keep information gathered from sensors intact, security and privacy are required at all the three layers discussed above for a healthcare framework [27].

2.7.4 Scalability

Information gathering in the healthcare systems nowadays focus on the use of sensors or health gadgets. These devices must be present in the entire clinic or building to benefit each and every patient to monitor their health records via their mobile devices. Moreover, for remote monitoring and consultation, these must be scalable up to an entire city or a region. The remote monitoring, diagnosis, consultation, and specialist recommendations would ultimately benefit patients by saving waiting time for appointments, avoiding long traveling times, and building a strong trust among patient and supervisors.

2.8 Conclusion

Real-time computation in critical situations is the basic requirement for any healthcare system. This chapter presented the concept of introducing an IFCL between the large IoT devices layer and the cloud. The introduction of IFN offered a real-time response delivery for delay-sensitive patient requests by use of its in-network caching capability. The smart health gateway performs intelligent computations to differentiate critical data from regular data. The migration from IP address to use of content naming has further contributed to optimal performance of the healthcare framework by addressing issues related to big data management, mobility, naming, and security. The highest benefit of adding ICN to healthcare is that it allows patients to get their requests processed at the node level and then to network with ease. The integration of ICN with fog has offered improved QoS with low latency and better network resources utilization.

References

1 Minaie, A., Sanati-Mehrizy, A., Sanati-Mehrizy, P., and Mehrizy, R.S. (2013). Application of wireless sensor networks in health care system. *Age* 23 (1).

2 Dohr, A., Modre-Opsrian, R., Drobics, M. et al. (2010). The internet of things for ambient assisted living. In: *2010 Seventh International Conference on Information Technology: New Generations*, 804–809. IEEE.

3 Miorandi, D., Sicari, S., De Pellegrini, F., and Chlamtac, I. (2012). Internet of things: vision, applications and research challenges. *Ad Hoc Networks* 10 (7): 1497–1516.

4 Koop, C.E., Mosher, R., Kun, L. et al. (2008). Future delivery of health care: cybercare. *IEEE Engineering in Medicine and Biology Magazine* 27 (6): 29–38.

5 Yousefpour, A., Fung, C., Nguyen, T. et al. (2019). All one needs to know about fog computing and related edge computing paradigms: a complete survey. *Journal of Systems Architecture* 98: 289–330.

6 Amadeo, M., Campolo, C., Quevedo, J. et al. (2016). Informationcentric networking for the internet of things: challenges and opportunities. *IEEE Network* 30 (2): 92–100.

7 Din, I.U., Hassan, S., Khan, M.K. et al. (2017). Caching in information-centric networking: strategies, challenges, and future research directions. *IEEE Communication Surveys and Tutorials* 20 (2): 1443–1474.

8 Arshad, S., Azam, M.A., Rehmani, M.H., and Loo, J. (2018). Recent advances in information-centric networking-based internet of things (ICN-IoT). *IEEE Internet of Things Journal* 6 (2): 2128–2158.

9 Amadeo, M., Campolo, C., Iera, A., and Molinaro, A. (2014). Nameddata networking for IoT: an architectural perspective. In: *2014 European Conference on Networks and Communications (EuCNC)*, 1–5. IEEE.

10 Aboodi, A., Wan, T.-C., and Sodhy, G.-C. (2019). Survey on the incorporation of NDN/CCN in IoT. *IEEE Access* 7: 71827–71858.

11 Zhang, Lixia, Deborah Estrin, Jeffrey Burke, Van Jacobson, James D. Thornton, Diana K. Smetters, Beichuan Zhang, Gene Tsudik, Dan Massey, and Christos Papadopoulos (2010)."Named data networking (ndn) project." Relat'orio T'ecnico NDN-0001, Xerox Palo Alto Research Center-PARC 157 (2010): 158.

12 Catarinucci, L., De Donno, D., Mainetti, L. et al. (2015). An IoT-aware architecture for smart healthcare systems. *IEEE Internet of Things Journal* 2 (6): 515–526.

13 Yeole, A.S. and Kalbande, D.R. (2016). Use of internet of things (IoT) in healthcare: a survey. In: *Proceedings of the ACM Symposium on Women in Research*, 71–76.2016

14 Sodhro, A.H., Luo, Z., Sangaiah, A.K., and Baik, S.W. (2019). Mobile edge computing based QoS optimization in medical healthcare applications. *International Journal of Information Management* 45: 308–318.

15 Farahani, B., Firouzi, F., Chang, V. et al. (2018). Towards fog-driven IoT eHealth: promises and challenges of IoT in medicine and healthcare. *Future Generation Computer Systems* 78: 659–676.

16 Sohn, S.Y., Bae, M., Lee, D.-k.R., and Kim, H. (2015). Alarmsystem for elder patients medication with IoT-enabled pill bottle. In: *2015 International Conference on Information and Communication Technology Convergence (ICTC)*, 59–61. IEEE.

17 Laranjo, I., Macedo, J., and Santos, A. (2012). Internet of things formedication control: service implementation and testing. *Procedia Technology* 5: 777–786.

18 Kalantarian, H., Motamed, B., Alshurafa, N., and Sarrafzadeh, M. (2016). Awearable sensor system for medication adherence prediction. *Artificial Intelligence in Medicine* 69: 43–52.

19 Rghioui, A., Sendra, S., Lloret, J., and Oumnad, A. (2016). Internetof things for measuring human activities in ambient assisted living and e-health. *Network Protocols and Algorithms* 8 (3): 15–28.

20 Lavanya, R. (2019). Fog computing and its role in the internet of things. In: *Advancing Consumer-Centric Fog Computing Architectures*, 63–71. IGI Global.

21 Dastjerdi, A.V. and Buyya, R. (2016). Fog computing: helping the internet of things realize its potential. *Computer* 49 (8): 112–116.

22 Vora, J., Tanwar, S., Tyagi, S. et al. (2017). FAAL: fog computing-based patient monitoring system for ambient assisted living. In: *2017 IEEE 19th International Conference on e-Health Networking, Applications and Services (Healthcom)*, 1–6. IEEE.

23 Vora, J., Tanwar, S., Tyagi, S. et al. (2017). Home-based exercise system for patients using IoT enabled smart speaker. In: *2017 IEEE 19th International Conference on e-Health Networking, Applications and Services (Healthcom)*, 1–6. IEEE.

24 Tasic, J., Gusev, M., and Ristov, S. (2016). A medical cloud. In: *2016 39th International Convention on Information and Communication Technology, Electronics and Microelectronics (MIPRO)*, 400–405. IEEE.

25 Aazam, M. and Huh, E.-N. (2015). E-HAMC: leveraging fog computing foremergency alert service. In: *2015 IEEE International Conference on Pervasive Computing and Communication Workshops (PerCom Workshops)*, 518–523. IEEE.

26 Anya, O. and Tawfik, H. (2017). Designing for practice-based contextawareness in ubiquitous e-health environments. *Computers and Electrical Engineering* 61: 312–326.

27 Mukherjee, M., Matam, R., Shu, L. et al. (2017). Security and privacy in fog computing: challenges. *IEEE Access* 5: 19293–19304.

3

Internet of Things (IoT) Enabled Software Defined Networking (SDN) for Load Balancing, Edge, Cloud Computing in Healthcare

Himanshi Babbar[1], Shalli Rani[1], and Neeraj Kumar[2]

[1] *Chitkara University Institute of Engineering and Technology, Chitkara University, Punjab, India*
[2] *Department of Computer Science and Engineering, Thapar University, Patiala, Punjab, India*

3.1 Overview of Software-Defined Networking

Software-defined networking (SDN) emerges as one of the noteworthy networking concepts which gives the hope to modify the limitations of current network infrastructures [1]. SDN has transposed the way of managing the network, and it is defined by two different tendencies: (i) SDN decouples the control level (controllers) from the data level (forwarding plane), and (ii) decoupling makes the control level programmable by the end users. In conventional networks, it is hardly possible to separate the control level from the data level [2]. Therefore, the end users had to be dependent on the merchants for the configuration of a software network and its users. This traditional network data plane informs your data where it is required to go, and the control plane is situated inside a switch or router, which could make the decision of progressing the packet and is also in charge of maintaining the routing table information and required to reserve the data; SDN was defined to design, build, and manage the networks that decouple the network layer and forwarding layer and is directly programmable by the source automation tools [3].

IoT-Enabled Smart Healthcare Systems, Services and Applications, First Edition.
Edited by Shalli Rani, Maheswar Rajagopal, Neeraj Kumar and Syed Hassan Ahmed Shah.

3.2 Overview of Healthcare

Throughout the healthcare industry, Wi-Fi networks are widely implemented, which improves the accessibility and reliability of services. The drawback to a large-scale deployment is the underlying security concerns that are highlighted because of the rise of wireless devices and the spontaneous deployment of access points (APs) [4]. A variety of repeated connections are required to achieve an optimized load-balancing state. The load-balancing decisions are made either by changing the APs' coverage area or by regulating the process of association regulation. Because of nonstatistical protocols and hardware, the load-balancing operations in conventional Wi-Fi networks are difficult to accomplish [5].

Hardware technological innovation and development have been incorporated. A new idea, Artificial Intelligence of Things (AIoT), was invented by the convergence of AI and IoT, where connected devices represent the digital nervous system and AI is a device's core. The AIoT enters the everyday activities of different industrial applications such as smart health, smart city, retail, and logistics. [6]. AIoT devices relay data for IoT devices in such technologies for decision-making, servers of the cloud via edge computing in healthcare. For instance, by offering healthcare services safely and effectively, a smart city application enhances the quality of life (QoL). After combining AI-enabled edge computing and disparate IoT-enabled networks to transfer medical data in an effective and timely way, AIoT-enabled health applications gained prominence. The resource-restricted existence of IoT devices and their stability are significant issues with many other IoT-based devices. As a result, through the safe and efficient use of enough resources of IoT devices, especially in healthcare, AIoT applications are becoming popular. As IoT devices constantly track patients in healthcare systems and constantly communicate the required data, they ought to be protected from malicious activities [4]. There are two basic issues with real-time monitoring and analysis of healthcare data: continuous and stable data transmission. Versatile authentication mechanisms are the best way to protect a low-powered IoT-enabled network.

To resolve these limitations, it is important to use versatile devices at the network edge, near the wearables, using edge computing, an authentication scheme, and data processing. A popular approach to building such a device is to provide the edge server with an intelligent SDN controller, which helps to achieve load balancing and effective use of resources.

3.2.1 How Software-Defined Networking (SDN) Is Benefitting Healthcare

In the never-ending goal to keep the standard of patient care, thus saving time and streamlining processes, healthcare innovations have played an important role for practitioners and facilities. Combined with wearable devices and other patient-centered technology, the IoT, big data, and real-time analytics have expanded patient care well beyond the four walls of conventional medical facilities and therefore have significantly improved diagnosis and treatment. Consequently, with fewer human errors, electronic health records (EHRs), digital imaging data, and pill dispensing systems are improving the quality of patient care.

However, in many instances, the rising role of technology in the medical field places a growing emphasis on the networks of healthcare providers. Health technology advances can often demand so much throughput that they slow down the capacity of the network, perhaps to the point of inefficiency or disruption of operations and patient care. In the meantime, healthcare providers are also continually concentrating on medical data protection in pursuit of new ways to deal with internal and external threats.

As a consequence, many businesses are continuing to update their infrastructure to meet the innovations that are rapidly at the forefront of healthcare. SDN may also be the gateway to help healthcare providers upgrade their networks and prevent disruption, continue to save money on network infrastructure, decrease network management complexity, improve security through added knowledge, and simplify compliance, among other advantages. The effects of data collection applications and significantly increased standards for connectivity are transforming the way networks are designed [7]. SDN helps to relieve the network's difficulty. There are many advantages, varying from versatility and cost savings to performance and safety. The advantages for providers of healthcare include:

- The SDN distinguishes network intelligence from data, allowing network administrators to control network devices from a single central location. Institutions can provide all their network services in all areas using an SDN controller, saving time and resources by decreasing the amount of manpower necessary at each facility.
- The network security often benefits from centralized management, with SDN controllers establishing an efficient central control point to execute policies. Fortunately, healthcare organizations will maintain their

networks, and the growing number of devices attached to them are protected and compatible by a centralized security control for all network devices. Another advantage is that administrators can differentiate network environments by adding another layer of protection for sensitive data, such as patient health records.
- Since SDN can centralize and optimize many repetitive network administration problems, healthcare organizations that implement it could save on manpower expenses. Central management ensures that tasks are performed more efficiently and with a reduced probability of error, thereby decreasing overhead network administration, particularly in multilocation organizations.
- The open-source design of SDN helps organizations, as all network intelligence lives at the controller, to minimize dependency on their current hardware. This not only helps to save money for organizations but also offers a straightforward migration road.

3.3 Technologies Used in Software-Defined Networking (SDN) and HealthCare

The technologies used in SDN healthcare are classified as described below in Figure 3.1.

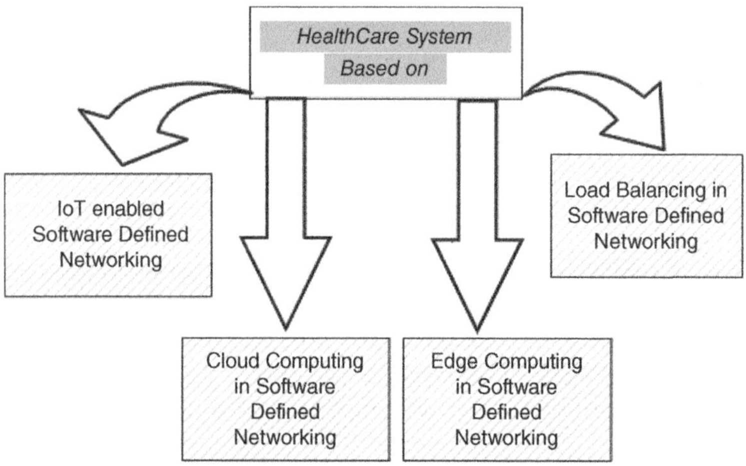

Figure 3.1 Technologies of SDN in healthcare.

3.3.1 Internet of Things in Software-Defined Networking

The two different available networking technologies are IoT and SDN. IoT consist primarily of sensing devices that comprise various communication networks, while SDN is concerned with network routing and functions as a network-level management orchestrator. SDN is a distinction between the control plane and the data plane, while IoT is a layered architecture and offers vendor independence [8]. It consists of various technologies at each level. Therefore, because SDN promises to keep the traditional network with new service requirements, IoT will leverage benefits from the SDN control plane.

3.3.1.1 Internet of Things (IoT)-Enabled Software-Defined Networking (SDN) in HealthCare

In recent decades, the population has increased dramatically, and this trend is projected to continue for many decades. This chapter, focused on the healthcare Internet of Things (HealthIoT), develops an emotionally immersive device with an intellectual framework based on cloud and body area networking (BAN) cross-network cooperation that can adequately interpret the user's physical and mental problems via wearable technology and BAN [9]. HealthIoT is also in its preliminary implementation stages. There is no chance, nevertheless, that the significance of HealthIoT will rise exponentially in upcoming everyday life, as has been the case with the Internet. While, in many ways, the Internet has accomplished tremendous success and improvements, it still faces issues. Intelligent control, on the one hand, is realized by different paths, and specifications and procedures are incorporated into every single router, making it hard to modify. Since the Internet's overall design is static, its growth is very slow. Besides, it makes technology infrastructure dynamic and error-prone based on the supplier's GUI [6]. But on the other side, this only provides best-effort service, so it inhibits the growth of highly specialized applications and does not fulfill unique service quality and user interface criteria.

The architecture of the HealthIoT framework must eliminate the above issues in the future to promote sustainable growth and encourage versatile management of diverse application requirements. According to the viewpoint of IoT evolution, the foregoing are some patterns that need to be addressed for the prospective HealthIoT development [7]. By distinguishing the control and data planes, SDN makes the adaptive network control feasible. SDN has indeed been applied to the mobile access network and 5th generation wireless network, guided by this benefit. In the IoT era, the physical infrastructure will become much more complicated, so it is critical

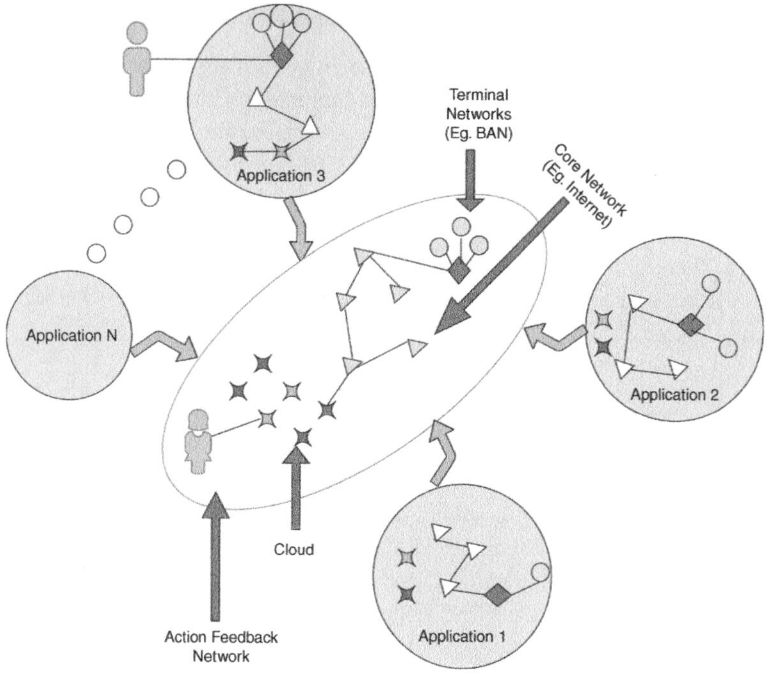

Figure 3.2 SDN-IoT based on healthcare network.

to achieve dynamic management and control of the IoT infrastructure via the SDN paradigm.

The development in distributing the basic infrastructure is the provision of the application programming interface (API) shown in Figure 3.2. Such APIs are supported by cloud suppliers such as Google APP Engine, and network controllers such as Floodlight also facilitate the northbound interface to create the application software for power [10]. To make physical infrastructure distribution feasible, an API often distinguishes the basic infrastructure's complexity and functional properties, which greatly decreases the challenge of designing the application software and reduces the time to market for the new app. This trend demonstrates that the IoT, particularly the sensor platform, must facilitate the application programmed with an API to flexibly and efficiently improve its capabilities. The figure illustrates this architecture's conceptual application [11]. The physical networks, BAN, sensor network, router, and remote cloud server are part of the basic infrastructure. Various health monitoring systems are implemented depending on that architecture, but each application customizes its own data set, delivery, and retrieval by the service interface.

Healthcare is moving to edge devices allowed by the IoT. Via a connection, edge devices are linked to one another. While there are many benefits to this, often there are also challenges. Hence the necessity for a network capable of controlling the complexities of having an IoT-enabled network [12]. One of the issues is important data about the health of every patient, so safety is one of the main concerns. Besides, this network can involve several networks as well. Therefore, if one is searching for medical records of patients from a connected IoT-enabled diagnostic imaging system, that requires the highest throughput from the device. The required network of hospitals, however, requires agility and versatility. Innovation in conventional networks and the ability to handle the following challenges are important.

- **Massive inputs of generated data:** Having thousands of devices in a single healthcare facility and a thousand more sending information from remote locations—all in real-time—will generate huge amounts of data. The data generated from IoT in healthcare will likely make storage requirements grow much higher, from terabytes to petabytes. If used properly, AI-driven algorithms and the cloud can help make sense of and organize this data, but this approach needs time to mature. So creating a large-scale IoT healthcare solution will take a lot of time and effort.
- **IoT devices will increase the attack surface:** IoT healthcare brings numerous benefits to the industry, but it also create numerous vulnerable security spots. Hackers could log into medical devices connected to the Internet and steal the information—or even modify it [12]. They can also take a step further and hack an entire hospital network, infecting the IoT devices with an infamous ransomware virus. That means the hackers will hold patients and their heart-rate monitors, blood pressure readers, and brain scanners as hostages.
- **Existing software infrastructure is obsolete:** IT infrastructures in many hospitals are obsolete. They will not allow for proper integration of IoT devices. Therefore, healthcare facilities will need to revamp their IT processes and use new, more modern software [13]. They will also need to take advantage of virtualization (technologies such as SDN and NFV, network function virtualization) and ultra-fast wireless and mobile networks such as advanced LTE or 5G.

3.3.2 Edge Computing

The edge computing concepts facilitate a more decentralized architecture where most mechanisms are carried out on the devices themselves. Edge computing uses a mesh network of relatively small data centers (DCs) rather than one centrally controlled center that can collect and manage data locally at the "edge" of the network. When edge computing and information security come, there are two opposite viewpoints: (i) it may assist to boost data security by storing, processing, and analyzing confidential information near the source rather than transmitting it over the network, and (ii) the risk exists that end devices could be much more resistant to threats than a centralized DC network.

3.3.2.1 e-Healthcare Edge Computing in Software-Defined Networking

The edge computing layer is made up of numerous SDN-based edge servers, which are capable of processing, storing, and collaborating with other servers for intellectual data. SDN-based edge computing aims to provide a variety of services, such as reduced latency, better performance, high scalability, and proximity services [13]. The SDN controller is designed in such a way that load balancing and optimum network architecture allow efficient use of resources. The SDN controller and all the details about storage, processing, and interaction functionality within every edge server are available together with incoming and outgoing traffic from IoT devices. The SDN controller defines cooperation between edge servers based on the load on all these servers and some predetermined guidelines. This method is achieved by cooperation between edge servers and efficient use of computer and storage resources.

Edge computing develops cloud computing (CC) as an efficient and convenient model. By attempting to bring computing resources close to the edge of an IoT-enabled network, it delivers low-latency cloud services. The goal is to reduce processing and traffic loads from low-powered IoT devices to efficient edge servers. In either way, load balancing is accomplished, resulting in decreased delays and support for mobility [14]. Economic growth and environmental changes have increased the mortality of chronic conditions, so that they are now the biggest danger to human health. It is possible for conventional healthcare systems to be divided into three layers, i.e., the compilation layer, the transmission layer, and the analysis layer. The device in the BAN gathers the sensed information at the fixed interval in the collection layer and delivers it through the smart terminal or smartphone to the gateway node or base station (BS), after which, via the Internet, the gateway or BS transfers it to the analysis layer (such as a cloud DC), and the data is stored and evaluated using machine learning and data mining algorithms in the cloud DC [15]. Finally, the device obtains the users' health status and takes the corresponding steps of medical care.

There are various factors in the healthcare system that have made healthcare more convenient for patients:

- Owing to the intra-modality of medical data, the conventional methods of machine learning and data mining struggle to uncover the hidden value in the data accurately. Thus, for a thorough disease analysis of all types of data, a more intellectual approach is needed.
- For processing, BAN sensors send the health data to the cloud, which enhances the access time of communication and neglects to offer immediate medical attention, analysis, and service in emergencies.
- The rigid implementation of network infrastructure results in a waste of time and resources. Besides, it does not provide users with a customized resource service for their various health statuses.

To overcome the above-mentioned issues, edge-based computing in smart healthcare systems arises. With edge computing, this scheme can collect and evaluate the physical health of users. In addition to a health risk assessment table [17], the existing framework acquires the corresponding health risk grade of the user under various health status updates, thus regulating the computing resource allocation of the entire edge computing network adequately according to each user's health risk grade and allowing the network to provide a user-oriented deeper cognitive application.

It is important to understand an intelligent and real-time healthcare system to implement the definite potential of cognitive computing on the edge of the network and carry out a cognitive examination of the physical health data and network resources of the client. This significantly eliminates latency and provides clients in an emergency with more contact resources and also provides the doctor with accurate and up-to-date patient information. Figure 3.3 demonstrates a healthcare system focused on the edge [18]. User 1 is connected to the edge node of Edge1, while users 2 and 3 are connected to the edge node of Edge1. The system accepts the scenario, then redistributes the resources, and allocates Edge1 to users 1, 2, and 3. The smart healthcare system built on the edge enables data cognition and cognition of capital, offering better energy efficiency, reduced cost, and high quality of experience (QoE) for patients. In detail, we will implement the edge-based healthcare, which includes the healthcare engine based on edge and the healthcare data flow form based also on edge.

In recent decades, edge computing has been effectively implemented and now is frequently used in various medical equipment. Edge computing allows end users to track and respond to health-related data created by multiple servers. To enjoy the benefits of collaborative computing paradigms,

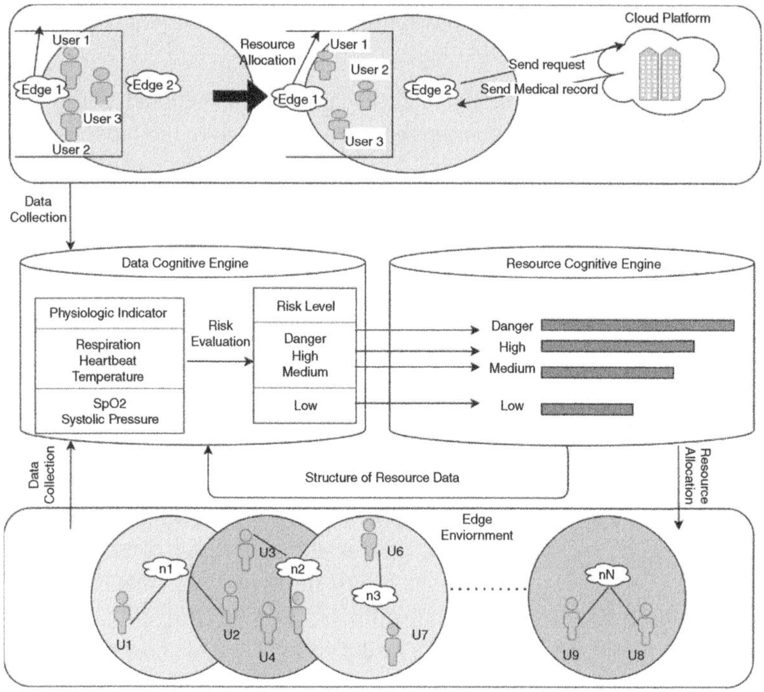

Figure 3.3 Edge based on SDN in e-healthcare.

various architectures that use cloud, SDN, and edge computing have been proposed. Healthcare applications are commonly known as delay-sensitive IoT applications [19]. Cloud computing was initially used for healthcare applications, but due to latency problems, it was not particularly successful. The implementation of edge computing solved these problems and made cloud computing practical for IoT applications in healthcare.

3.3.3 Cloud Computing in Software-Defined Networking

Cloud computing is an essential software technology based on the idea of lower expenditure and pay-per-use billing options, with pay-as-you-go models generally used by cloud service providers. As this model offers a natural match for a broad range of applications, such as those that exploit the capacity of the IoT domain, the implementation of cloud-based services is becoming more and more widespread. In computer networking, SDN is a network architecture approach wherein network administrators can handle network services via flexible control and functions specified by the software. For easy handling, the SDN definition implies the separation of network control functions from its data plane and enables remote access to the network traffic control switches in the DC. This sets it apart from traditional concepts of network management. In software-defined cloud computing (SDCC), SDN principles are essential because they promote multi-tiered applications and guarantee that user transactions are performed within certain service level agreements within a specified time frame.

3.3.3.1 e-Healthcare Software-Defined Networking in Cloud Computing with Wireless Body Area Networks (WBANs)

Cloud computing (CC) has been one of the new technologies that offer a virtual network with unprecedented versatility in computing, storage, and software services. Thousands of server clusters and storage centers as well as other virtual server resources can be handled by the cloud at a minimal price [19]. The virtualized computational resource pool that could measure and extend to even more computational resources can be represented as cloud computing. The networking infrastructure is now becoming complicated and difficult to maintain as technologies grow over time. For all of that, a new concept arose for a mathematical and memory-intensive operation of network management, which also brings support to improve the shortcomings of the present network infrastructure. This type of concept is called software-defined networking (SDN). The dominant aspect of SDN is to disassociate the control plane from the data plane [20], which makes the configuration of the network easier.

In the **SDN-data plane**, the data packets are forwarded by each network interface in accordance with the policies that have been configured on that system, and in the **SDN-control plane** the controller is managed for configuring and controlling the network behavior of the rules on the devices of the network. To more efficiently control operations and take the burden off network hardware, healthcare organizations are incorporating health IT technology using virtualization [21] and making IT systems more simplified and flexible; more organizations also use SDN solutions. Research and market analysts forecast that, due to the need to make IT systems smaller and simpler to manage, the SDN market will grow at a CAGR of 40% by 2024. By the study, healthcare is described as one of the verticals most likely to implement SDN technology. Networks must be able to accommodate the increasing volume of traffic as healthcare institutions transition to EHRs and cloud computing. Therefore, to achieve enhanced network flexibility and visibility, companies are adopting cloud-based healthcare SDN solutions. These technologies can also assist organizations to make better use of the cloud for medical resources and applications. By centralizing managerial functions into a server computer that determines how data travels across the network, SDN eliminates the complications of wireless hardware [23]. This enables IT administrators to maintain more control over their networks and to respond more quickly to network demands. SDN uses virtualization to isolate network hardware from intelligent management software. And thereby, SDN establishes a network model that is centralized, more intelligent, and more easily controlled.

As an essential technology for decentralized healthcare systems and also the virtual hospitalization market, wireless body area networks (WBANs) have gained prominence. Used mostly for WBANs, miniaturized wearable devices can capture critical signals and gestures and can transfer them to dedicated medical servers. Since cloud computing has benefits in terms of usability, flexibility, and cost effectiveness, it may be a stronger option to take advantage of these benefits. WBANs incorporation. Besides, SDN, renowned as an evolving architecture, could add another dimension to cloud computing in terms of adaptability, high capacity for bandwidth, and manageability. As various mobile healthcare system applications become prevalent day by day and medical video streaming becomes a primary concern, in terms of quality of service (QoS) and other functionalities, cloud computing allows SDN to be part of solution to this issue.

3.3.3.2 Benefits of SDN with Cloud Computing in WBANs

i) **Managing the data:** The consistent information gathered by the WBAN detectors must be effectively accumulated, processed, and stored [24]. In terms of computation, the database management system has to be dispersed. This management system could be facilitated by cloud computing by allowing fast and efficient access to a huge scale of storage.

ii) **Evaluate and analyze the data:** The information gathered can be acquired for evaluation and analysis of the medical decision-making based on the medical decision management (MDM) scheme.

iii) **Management of centralized system:** With the assistance of SDN controllers that retain a reliable network, the network information can be centralized by the use of SDN in networking. Besides that, the QoS function can be configured using OpenFlow.

3.3.4 Load Balancing in Software-Defined Networking

Load balancing is defined as the distribution of load among the different servers to optimize the resources, decrease the response time, and increase the throughput. In the conventional load-balancing networks, it facilitates the support of hardware that is very expensive and suffers from a lack of flexibility; with this it becomes a single point of failure easily. Availability of service is predominant in aligning the satisfaction of the end users, which has a higher level of significance on the achievement of balancing the load among the process clusters. The connection of most of the people with the Internet affects the web traffic, which causes the congestion of the network and the loss of packets. With this technique, load balancing optimizes the efficiency of the network.

3.3.4.1 e-Healthcare Load Balancing in Software-Defined Networking

To improve the accessibility and reliability of services, Wi-Fi networks are widely used in the healthcare industry [25]. The drawback to this immense-scale development is the underlying issues that are heightened due to the rise in wireless devices and the spontaneous implementation of APs. To achieve an optimum load-balancing state, a variety of repeated connections are required. The load balancing decisions are made either by changing the APs' network coverage or by regulating the process of connection regulation. Due to the lack of standardized regulations and hardware, the load-balancing tasks in conventional Wi-Fi networks are difficult to accomplish.

SDN is a new methodology, which, by distinguishing the control plane from the data plane, serves as a means of organizing network functions. In the management of the network and control tasks, this separation offers simplicity [21]. A centralized view of the entire network enables intelligent forwarding decisions to be made by the SDN controller. Rather than depending on hardware customized and designs of protocol, we assume that the combination of SDN and Wi-Fi, i.e., software-defined Wi-Fi networks (SD-Wi-Fi), will produce better load-balancing techniques. In this section, we have discussed the traffic-aware load balancing technique in healthcare.

The system architecture in Figure 3.4 comprises a centralized controller, APs, web servers, and Wi-Fi stations activated by OpenFlow. On obtaining the status reports of APs, the controller measures the fairness index of the JAIN and computes the average load age for wise decisions on balancing the load. The server-based application hosts a range of other servers, comprised of file servers, multimedia servers, servers for web applications, and so forth. These servers acknowledge requests from users on the Wi-Fi network. Balancing the load and applications based on traffic awareness running on the SDN controller guarantees that even the distribution of load among the APs is accomplished and the traffic that is delay-sensitive such as an electrocardiogram is assigned high priority.

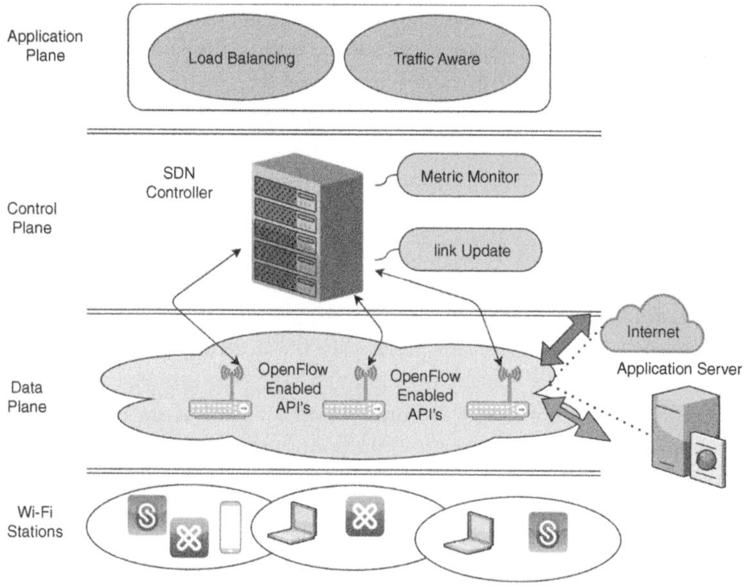

Figure 3.4 Architecture of load balancing in SDN healthcare.

3.4 Use Cases of Software-Defined Networking in Healthcare

Networking is becoming more dynamic in today's new technology, such as cloud computing and the IoT. Stable connectivity may be an obstacle to having adequate bandwidth in real time. This is also particularly relevant in healthcare, where protection, compliance, and patient safety all enhance the privacy and scalability of data transfer [24]. This is why in health information technology most healthcare organizations are exploring SDN solutions along with cloud and edge.

- **Prioritization of network traffic:** In a situation where the reliability of a network will affect the life or death of a patient, healthcare organizations must have substantial exposure to network facilities that prioritize smart traffic. For example, the network appears to be able to explain the difference between a doctor who wants to access annual check-up documents or one who accesses others for immediate surgery. The use of SDN in health IT helps ensure that the least important traffic seldom takes priority over transmitting hospital records to everyone in an emergency room, along with such back-office applications or an executive watching YouTube in the hospital canteen.

- **Decreasing error instances:** These are among the key benefits of using SDN to boost network management by automating the synchronization of packets on various routes. In a traditional network setup, the acquisition of infrastructure is one of the most time-consuming areas of IT.
- **Track configuration changes:** Whether a change has been made dynamically or by a system administrator, configuration adjustments can be easily identified via SDN. If proactive control is required in the event of an error, the activities can be more focused because each change is logged.
- **Ideally suited for mergers and acquisitions:** In ancient times, the introduction of a new acquisition or merger into the existing network created many problems. It takes a few days to integrate a new site into the network with SDN in health IT introducing limit-touch procurement.
- **Patient monitoring:** Patient monitoring requires an effective, scalable, versatile, safe monitoring system that requires the provision of patient information anywhere in a hospital. Patient monitoring is allowed when they travel from one location to another to look ahead to the patients. Besides, a wire can be plugged into an open port to create a network loop. Contemporary medical monitoring endpoints support both wired and wireless features and stable communication of the monitoring system controller as it differs between wired and wireless connections. If an endpoint monitoring a patient joins the network, it is detected by an SDN controller. In general, the system switches information to pass and forward, allowing the endpoint to communicate directly with the medical monitoring controller. Any location within the network of SDN switches can be connected to the monitored network. An endpoint is specified by the SDN controller, and the virtual network interface is enabled.
- **Information security:** Until the modern era, patients would have to record their medical history. Fortunately, with the advent of electronic medical records, doctors may access a patient's medical details directly to prescribe medications and verify the results of the examination. Although electronic records offer various benefits for both doctors and patients, safety issues have been raised. Patient records need to be kept confidential, particularly with the rise of cyber threats [25]. SDN will provide the necessary security and flexibility to transfer patient data from one end point to another. For health-related web technologies, SDN controller technology can create virtual networks and install security systems tailored to any system. Also, Neelam Hospital has been approved to build four different virtual networks over a single network connection using SDN. By growing its 3G network, the hospital vowed to keep track of patients diagnosed.

- **Effective interaction:** For healthcare, it is critical that doctor and patient can see and talk to each other. They allow physicians to hold video conferences with patients, eliminating needless hours in waiting rooms. For patients living in rural areas who are unable to leave their homes for some reason, this is particularly useful. Medical services go further than the walls of hospitals with that kind of equipment. To provide such services, healthcare professionals need consistent and efficient contact and adequate QoS. For wired and wireless mobiles, static voice call implementations can work well [17]. SDN helps to inform the video or voice call network that is configured for the call itself by the successful communication controller.
- **Information exchange:** To avoid unnecessary duplication of laboratory tests, data sharing is critical in healthcare. As it can be obtained from various demographics, diagnoses, and medical records, this healthcare data can also be used for research purposes.

Figure 3.5 has projected that healthcare applications will increase in 2022since it has partnered with many other innovations, such as AI and the

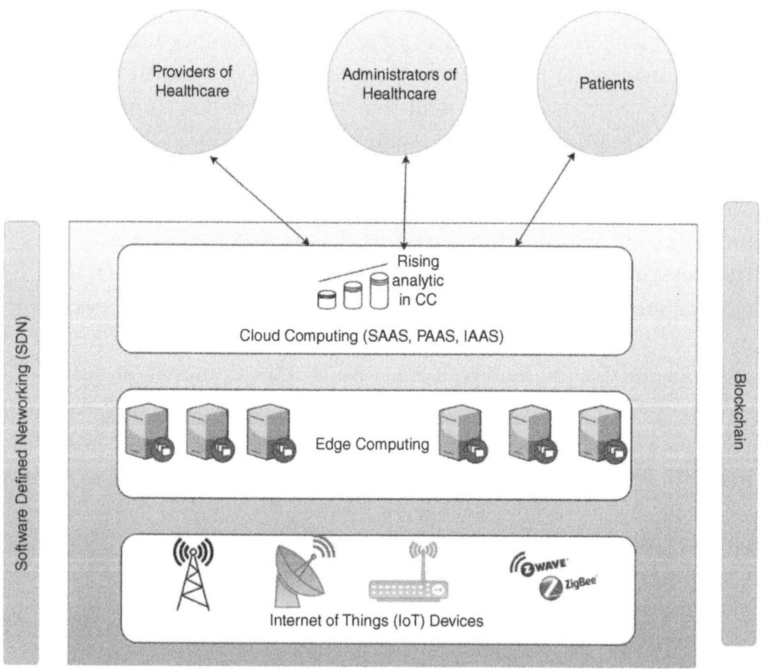

Figure 3.5 Software-defined networking in healthcare.

IoT. The partnership would support various stakeholders, such as NGOs, clinics, laboratories, hospitals, pharmaceutical firms, and supply chains. Healthcare is an essential method that stores and maintains patients' medical records [18]. This approach offers improved treatment, well-managed disease monitoring and causation, medical records for research purposes, and so forth. Hospitals are responsible for this data production. Diagnosing a condition is very challenging for healthcare workers and laboratory tests often need to be repeated, which is very challenging for patients. Different client-server or cloud-based healthcare systems are vulnerable to data fragmentation, protection, and privacy issues.

3.5 Research Directions

The relationship between cloud and edge computing appears to be an exciting architecture involving SDN as its driving force. The preceding report describes the developments in SDN and its experimental conditions that are highly feasible for the edge computing paradigm's hidden ability to be leveraged. Because both edge computing and SDN have not yet achieved the full level of their ability, the technology consisting of these innovative concepts may not live up to expectations and may not produce the intended efficiency. This naivety includes a variety of variables, but perhaps the most relevant ones are:

i) Requirements are rapidly changing; even the cloud-based comparatively more traditional domains such as IaaS (infrastructure as a service) are evolving.
ii) Specifications are becoming complex.
iii) Integrating SDN into existing networks is not easily accomplished by merely installing networking devices that are SDN-enabled.
iv) Hardware investments are costly, so SDN-enabled hardware does not meet the necessary level in terms of capability and deployment.

3.6 Conclusion

In this chapter we have described the development of the flexible HealthIoT framework, which interacts with both intelligent health monitoring and psychological treatment. Primarily, by distinguishing the application from the underlying physical infrastructure, we suggest a HealthIoT platform with software-specified capabilities. This addresses the issues of data redundancy and service response delay in the edge-cloud network based on

SDN. With this architecture, healthcare systems can be tailored with well-defined APIs to view their data collection, distribution, storage, and emotion input and access different applications to operate in a shared infrastructure to decrease the cost of capital and maintenance. We have thereby discussed the technologies benefitting and challenges on how SDN-IoT, edge, load balancing, and cloud computing can help healthcare organizations to enhance the reliability and accessibility of services and various benefits and challenges faced so that Wi-Fi networks are widely used in the healthcare industry.

Key Points

i) Software-defined networking (SDN) emerges as one of the noteworthy networking concepts, which gives the hope to modify the limitations of current network infrastructures.
ii) Hardware technological innovation and development have enabled real-time decision-making to be incorporated.
iii) Artificial Intelligence of Things (AIoT) was invented by the convergence of AI and IoT, where devices of IoT metaphorize the nervous system digitally and AI represents the system's brain.
iv) There are two basic issues with real-time monitoring and analysis of healthcare data: continuous and stable data transmission. Versatile authentication mechanisms are the best way to protect a low-powered IoT-enabled network.
v) Healthcare Internet of Things (HealthIoT) develops an emotionally immersive device with an intellectual framework based on cloud and BAN cross-network.
vi) The architecture of the HealthIoT framework must eliminate the above issues in the future to promote sustainable growth and encourage versatile management of diverse application requirements.
vii) By distinguishing the control and data planes, SDN allows adaptive network control.
viii) SDN uses virtualization to isolate network hardware from intelligent management software.
ix) SDN-based edge computing aims to provide a variety of services, such as minimized response time, enhanced performance, high scalability, and proximity services.
x) Collaboration between edge servers is determined by the SDN controller based on the load on these servers and some predetermined guidelines.
xi) The goal is to reduce processing and traffic loads from minimal-powered devices of IoT to efficient edge servers.

xii) The smart healthcare system built on the edge enables data cognition and cognition of capital, offering better energy efficiency, minimized cost, and enhanced patient's quality of experience (QoE).

xiii) SDN is a new methodology, which, by distinguishing the control plane from the data plane, serves as a means of organizing network functions. In the management of the network and control tasks, this separation offers simplicity.

xiv) Networking is becoming more dynamic in today's new technology, such as cloud computing and the IoT. Stable connectivity may be an obstacle to having adequate bandwidth in real time.

xv) The key benefit of using SDN is to boost network management by automating the synchronization of packets on various routes.

xvi) Healthcare is an essential method that stores and maintains patients' medical records. This approach offers improved treatment, well-managed disease monitoring and causation, medical records for research purposes, and so forth.

xvii) The preceding report describes the developments in SDN and its experimental conditions that are highly feasible for the edge computing paradigm's hidden ability to be leveraged.

Author Biography

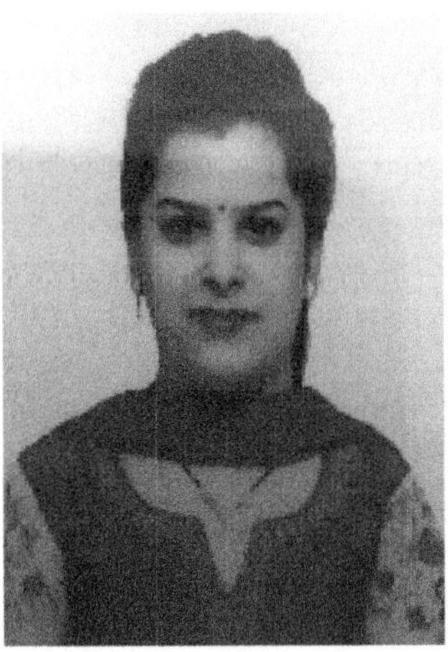

Ms. Himanshi Babbar is assistant professor and researcher in computer applications, working in Chitkara University, Rajpura, Punjab, India. She has two years of teaching experience at CGC, Landran, Mohali, Punjab. She completed an MCA (master's in computer applications) from Chitkara University, Punjab Campus, and is currently Pursuing a PhD in computer applications from Chitkara University, Punjab Campus. Her area of research is software-defined networking, load balancing, and the Internet of Things. She has attended six national conferences, published many papers in national and international journals, and filed 8 patents.

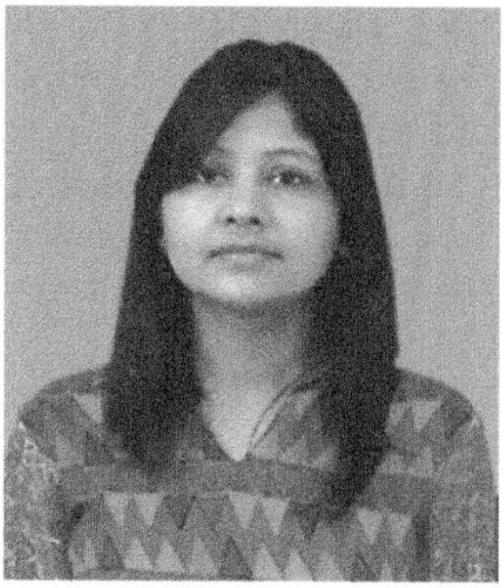

Ms. Shalli Rani is associate professor in CSE with Chitkara University, Rajpura, Punjab, India. She has 14+ years of teaching experience. She received an MCA degree from Maharishi Dayanand University, Rohtak, in 2004, an M.Tech. degree in computer science from Janardan Rai Nagar Vidyapeeth University, Udaipur, in 2007 and a PhD degree in computer applications from Punjab Technical University, Jalandhar, in 2017. Her main area of interest and research is wireless sensor networks, underwater sensor networks, and the Internet of Things. She has published and presented more than 25 papers in international journals and conferences. She has worked on big data, underwater acoustic sensors, and IoT to show the importance of WSN in IoT applications. She received a young scientist award in February 2014 from Punjab Science Congress, in the same field.

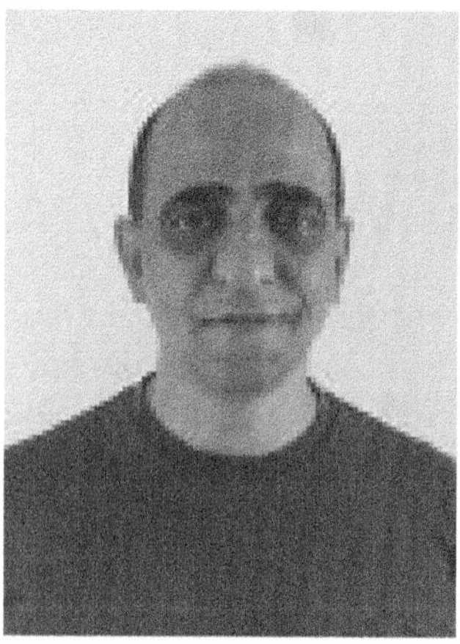

Mr. Neeraj Kumar is a full professor in the Department of Computer Science and Engineering, Thapar Institute of Engineering and Technology, Patiala (Pb.), India. He is also adjunct professor at Asia University, Taiwan, King Abdul Aziz University, Jeddah, Saudi Arabia, and Charles Darwin University, Australia. He has published more than 400 technical research papers (DBLP: https://dblp.org/pers/hd/k/Kumar_0001:Neeraj) in top-cited journals and conferences which are cited more than 17000 times from well-known researchers across the globe with current h-index of 71 (Google scholar: https://scholar.google.com/citations?hl=en&user=gL9gR-4AAAAJ). He has been a highly cited researcher in 2019 and 2020 in the list released by Web of Science (WoS). He has guided many research scholars leading to PhDs and M.E./M.Techs. His research is supported by funding from various competitive agencies across the globe. His broad research areas are green computing and network management, IoT, big data analytics, deep learning, and cyber security. He has also edited/authored 10 books with international/national publishers such as IET, Springer, Elsevier, and CRC: *Security and Privacy of Electronic Healthcare Records: Concepts, Paradigms and Solutions* (ISBN-13: 978-1-78561-898-7), *Machine Learning for Cognitive IoT*, CRC Press, *Blockchain, Big Data and Machine learning*, CRC Press, *Blockchain Technologies across Industrial Vertical*, Elsevier, *Multimedia Big Data Computing for IoT Applications: Concepts, Paradigms and Solutions* (ISBN: 978-981-13-8759-3), *Proceedings of First International Conference on Computing, Communications, and Cyber-Security* (IC4S 2019) (ISBN 978-981-15-3369-3). *Probabilistic Data Structures for Blockchain based IoT Applications*, CRC Press. One of the edited textbooks entitled, *Multimedia Big Data Computing for IoT Applications: Concepts, Paradigms, and Solutions*, published in Springer in 2019, has had 3.5 million downloads as of June 2020. It attracts the attention of researchers across the globe. (https://www.springer.com/in/book/9789811387586).

He has served as editor of *ACM Computing Survey*, *IEEE Transactions on Sustainable Computing*, *IEEE Systems Journal*, *IEEE Network Magazine*, *IEEE Communication Magazine*, *Elsevier Journal of Networks and Computer Applications*, *Elsevier Computer Communication*, *Wiley International Journal of Communication Systems*. Also, he has organized various special issues of journals of repute from IEEE, Elsevier, and Springer. He has been a workshop chair at IEEE Globecom 2018, IEEE Infocom 2020 (https://infocom2020.ieee-infocom.org/workshop-blockchain-secure-software-defined-networking-smart-communities) and IEEE ICC 2020 (https://icc2020.ieee-icc.org/workshop/ws-06-secsdn-secure-and-dependable-software-defined-networking-sustainable-smart) and track chair of Security and privacy of IEEE MSN 2020 (https://conference.cs.cityu.edu.hk/msn2020/cf-wkpaper.php). He is also TPC chair and member of various international conferences such as IEEE MASS 2020, IEEE MSN2020. He has won the best papers award from IEEE Systems Journal and IEEE ICC 2018, Kansas City in 2018. He won the best researcher award from parent organization every year for the last eight consecutive years.

References

1 Khayat, M., Barka, E., and Sallabi, F. (2019). SDN_based secure healthcare monitoring system (SDN-SHMS). In: *2019 28th International Conference on Computer Communication and Networks (ICCCN)*, 1–7.

2 Chakravarthy, V.D. and Amutha, B. (2020). Software-defined network-assisted packet scheduling method for load balancing in mobile user concentrated cloud. *Computer Communications* 150: 144–149.

3 Li, J., Cai, J., Khan, F. et al. (2020). A secured framework for SDN-based edge computing in IoT-enabled healthcare system. *IEEE Access* 8: 135479–135490.
4 Manzoor, S., Chen, Z., Gao, Y. et al. (2020). Towards QoS-aware load balancing for high-density software-defined Wi-Fi networks. *IEEE Access* 8: 117623–117638.
5 Baktir, A.C., Ozgovde, A., and Ersoy, C. (2017). How can edge computing benefit from software-defined networking: a survey, use cases, and future directions. *IEEE Communication Surveys and Tutorials* 19 (4): 2359–2391.
6 Manzoor, S., Karmon, P., Hei, X., and Cheng, W. (2020). Traffic aware load balancing in software-defined WiFi networks for healthcare. In: *2020 Information Communication Technologies Conference (ICTC)*, 81–85.
7 Baktir, A.C., Tunca, C., Ozgovde, A. et al. (2018). SDN-based multi-tier computing and communication architecture for pervasive healthcare. *IEEE Access* 6: 56765–56781.
8 Babbar, H. and Rani, S. (2019). Emerging prospects and trends in software defined networking. *Journal of Computational and Theoretical Nanoscience* 16 (10): 4236–4241.
9 Hasan, K., Ahmed, K., Biswas, K. et al. (2020). Control plane optimization for an SDN-based WBAN framework to support healthcare applications. *Sensors 20* (15): 4200.
10 Liu, Y., Zeng, Z., Liu, X. et al. (2019). A novel load balancing and low response delay framework for edge-cloud networks based on SDN. *IEEE Internet of Things Journal* 7 (7): 5922–5933.
11 Chen, M., Li, W., Hao, Y. et al. (2018). Edge cognitive computing-based smart healthcare system. *Future Generation Computer Systems* 86: 403–411.
12 Li, G., Wang, X., and Zhang, Z. (2019). SDN-based load balancing scheme for multi-controller deployment. *IEEE Access* 7: 39612–39622.
13 Abdelltif, A.A., Ahmed, E., Fong, A.T. et al. (2018). SDN-based load balancing service for cloud servers. *IEEE Communications Magazine* 56 (8): 106–111.
14 Gupta, S., Acharya, H.B., and Kwon, M. (2019). On securing healthcare with software-defined networks. In: *IEEE INFOCOM 2019-IEEE Conference on Computer Communications Workshops (INFOCOM WKSHPS)*, 354–359. IEEE.
15 Babbar, H. and Rani, S. (2020). Software-defined networking framework securing internet of things. In: *Integration of WSN and IoT for Smart Cities*, 1–14.
16 Babbar, H., Rani, S., Masud, M., Verma, S., Anand, D. and Jhanjhi, N., Load Balancing Algorithm for Migrating Switches in Software-Defined Vehicular Networks, *Computers, Materials and continua* 67(1): 1301–1316.

17 Zemrane, H., Baddi, Y., and Hasbi, A. (2019). Improve IoT eHealth ecosystem with SDN. In: *Proceedings of the 4th International Conference on Smart City Applications*, 1–8.

18 Aujla, G.S., Chaudhary, R., Kaur, K. et al. (2018). SAFE: SDN-assisted framework for anedge–cloud interplay in the secure healthcare ecosystem. *IEEE Transactions on Industrial Informatics* 15 (1): 469–480.

19 Bhatt, C.M. and Peddoju, S.K. (eds.) (2016). *Cloud Computing Systems and Applications in Healthcare*. IGI Global.

20 Hossain, M.S., Xu, C., Li, Y. et al. (2018). Advances in next-generation networking technologies for smart healthcare. *IEEE Communications Magazine* 56 (4): 14–15.

21 Sallabi, F., Naeem, F., Awad, M., and Shuaib, K. (2018). Managing IoT-based smart healthcare systems traffic with software-defined networks. In: *2018 International Symposium on Networks, Computers and Communications (ISNCC)*, 1–6. IEEE.

22 Shayokh, M.A., Kim, J.W., and Shin, S.Y. (2015). Cloud-based software-defined wireless body area networks architecture for the virtual hospital. In: *Proceedings of the 10th EAI International Conference on Body Area Networks*, 92–95.

23 Benzekki, K., El Fergougui, A., and Elbelrhiti Elalaoui, A. (2016). Software-defined networking (SDN): a survey. *Security and Communication Networks* 9 (18): 5803–5833.

24 Fernandez, F. and Pallis, G.C. (2014). Opportunities and challenges of the internet of things for healthcare: systems engineering perspective. In: *2014 4th International Conference on Wireless Mobile Communication and Healthcare-Transforming Healthcare Through Innovations in Mobile and Wireless Technologies (MOBIHEALTH)*, 263–266. IEEE.

25 Devadass, L., Sekaran, S.S., and Thinakaran, R. (2017). Cloud computing in healthcare. *International Journal of Students' Research in Technology & Management* 5 (1): 25–31.

4

Security and Privacy Issues in Smart Healthcare System Using Internet of Things

R. Nidhya[1], Manish Kumar[2], R. Maheswar[3], and D. Pavithra[4]

[1] *Department of Computer Science and Engineering, Madanapalle Institute of Technology & Science, Madanapalle, Andhra Pradesh, India*
[2] *School of Computer Science and Engineering, Vellore Institute of Technology, Chennai, Tamil Nadu, India*
[3] *Dean Research (Assistant), VIT Bhopal University, Bhopal, India*
[4] *Department of Electronics and Communication Engineering, Sri Ramakrishna Institute of Technology, Coimbatore, Tamil Nadu, India*

4.1 Introduction

With the increasing growth of wireless communication and wearable sensors, the various smart developments to handle the real-world problems especially in smart healthcare (SHC) systems such as mobile wireless sensor networks (MWSNs) are proposed for real-time monitoring of the patients' health [1]. To monitor the motions and vital health parameters of a patient, sensors are being attached to garments or wearable devices. The gathered patients' health information is transmitted to the healthcare database. Healthcare providers will access the health data from the database for further investigation of a patient's health condition. Even a medical database may be shared with insurance companies, researchers, patients, or government agencies in case of any emergency or needed clarification regarding patient's health. In the same way medical emergency handling and clinical diagnosis has been developed to improve the effectiveness of healthcare, this will modernize the healthcare services provided to the patients and healthcare centers. A smart healthcare environment aims at providing a platform to the patients and practitioners to make available healthcare services flawlessly. MWSN when transmitting the data over the

IoT-Enabled Smart Healthcare Systems, Services and Applications, First Edition.
Edited by Shalli Rani, Maheswar Rajagopal, Neeraj Kumar and Syed Hassan Ahmed Shah.

Internet is also a part of Internet of Things (IoT). In an emergency, patients can be monitored remotely while healthcare providers share health information in real time [2].

The IoT is the internetworking of physical devices embedded with sensors, actuators, and network connectivity to make the device smart. These embedded devices can gather and forward the data to make a device connected and smart. By using the existing network, an IoT device can be controlled, which will provide an opportunity for direct computer-controlled devices to increase their efficiency and precision. This also results in economic benefits to the users. Nowadays, IoT connects the sensors and a massive number of devices with the Internet using IP-based communications. In healthcare applications, IoT provides various major features such as options to remote healthcare monitoring, emergency handling, elderly monitoring, early prevention, and medical treatment for the disabled. The collected IoT data are stored in the cloud for easy accessibility. The cloud-based smart healthcare (SHC) systems play a vital role in everyday life. Recently medical care takers store and retrieve patient health data in electronic health records (EHRs). Traditional paper systems are replaced by EHRs which will enhance the efficiency in the storage and retrieval of patients' health data [3–5]. EHRs are storing highly confidential personal data of patients in the cloud and are exchanged over the Internet and are therefore vulnerable to attacks [6–8], such as data misinterpretation, loss, and hacking. Nowadays, many cloud health data leaks have caught researchers' attention. Data privacy and security are indispensable attributes of an EHR-based healthcare system. Data security deals with storing and transferring the data securely to assure its validity, integrity, and authenticity. Data privacy deals with people who can access the data. There is significant ongoing research addressing these problems [9–13]. This chapter focuses on privacy and security issues of IoT in healthcare applications.

4.2 Overview of Internet of Things in Smart Healthcare Systems

There are plenty of methods to set up a smart healthcare system using IoT. The deployment of SHC in real-time applications depends on requirements such as the number of users, sensor network topology, and resources availability. The SHC is mostly client-server architecture. As shown in Figure 4.1, there are three major layers in the SHC system architecture. The first one is the sensor data acquisition layer deployed in real-time environment, which is used to gather the patient's healthcare information. To store

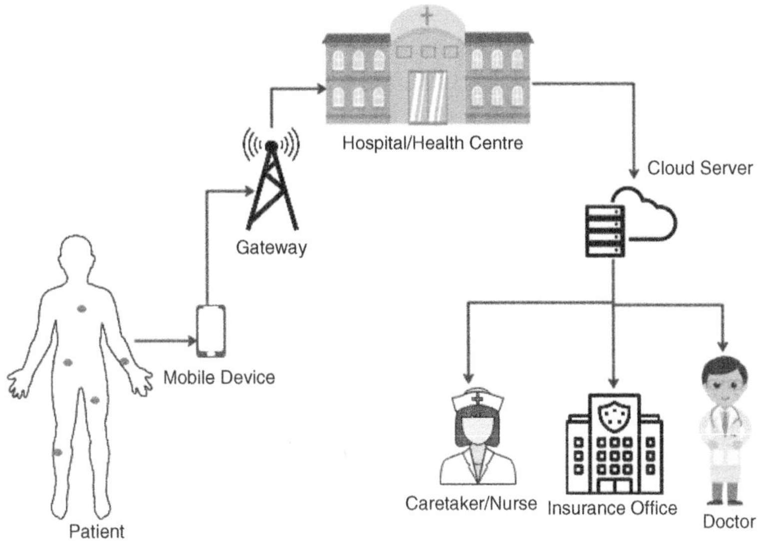

Figure 4.1 Architecture of Smart HealthCare System (SHC).

the data received from a patient, the data center, also called server, is deployed in the cloud. The healthcare information is transmitted from clients to server using the secure links [14]. The healthcare data acquisition layer consists of a field control unit and sensors, which are used to monitor body vital parameters such as blood pressure, blood sugar, brain activity, and heart rate. Field control units are responsible for controlling and managing heterogeneous data received from healthcare sensors, incorporate the received data, and convert it into an integrated homogeneous format. It also performs the preliminary data analysis according to the aggregate data's predefined format.

The data received from sensors will be transferred to the field control unit through wired or wireless transmission. Then the field control unit is connected to a medical cloud data server over the Internet by wired or wireless mode such as Bluetooth, Zigbee, Wi-Fi, Mobile network, or Li-Fi. to forward the health data. The major tasks of the cloud server are storing, managing, and security protection of the data. Data storage comprises different types of data such as video, image, semi-structured, unstructured, or structured. Implementation of data indexing, data fusion, analysis and displaying of data, and so forth will be handled by data management. Data security protection deals with health data encryption, audit logs, accessing authority management, data isolation, backup recovery, and so on. The architecture of IoT in healthcare integrated with cloud computing is shown in Figure 4.1. This helps to extensively advance healthcare-related services and present a better platform for uninterrupted and efficient innovation. IoT's healthcare simplifies the medical processes and improves the quality of healthcare services. Another use of IoT in healthcare is wearable healthcare devices or mobile healthcare applications, which permit patients to monitor their health information. Most of these are connected to devices such as mobiles, laptop, tablets, and handheld devices for empowering human lives. The collected data from electronic devices (imaging device, handheld device) are analyzed, which will improve the decision-making control. This makes the patients to focus more in their personal health management.

Since there are plenty of wireless healthcare devices interconnected to web-based communication systems, they become more vulnerable to attacks. This vulnerability occurs not only due to malicious attackers but also from multiple threats such as computer viruses, malware, and Trojan horses. Most of the healthcare organizations don't expend sufficient resources to provide security and privacy to their healthcare data. But security and privacy plays a major role in medical data. Healthcare devices are producing the vast amounts of heterogeneous real-time data for remote health monitoring of patients, which are highly sensitive in nature. Privacy in patient health information should exist in all levels of data collection, transmission, cloud storage, and so forth. While developing security and privacy systems for medical data transmission over the Internet, four mandatory requirements should be considered: data integrity, data usability, data privacy, and patient information privacy. Still there are a few more requirements to be considered to develop a more secure environment. They are data availability, data authentication, data notarization, data confidentiality, data unlinkability, data anonymity, data pseudonymity, data untraceability, data unobservability, and so forth.

4.3 Policies and Legislation Related to Smart Healthcare

The United States endorsed the rules and regulations for the implementation smart healthcare systems. The National Institute of Science and Technology (NIST) of the United States provided recommendations for different types of security controls imposed on smart healthcare environments, which are also applicable and relevant to the global implementation [15]. Specifically, NIST mentioned that any organization or government can adopt the standards suggested by them for risk management and security control mechanisms. A detailed view on various rules and regulations is provided in this section.

4.3.1 HIPAA in Privacy Rule

In 1996, the Health Insurance and Portability Accountability Act (HIPAA) [16] was and summarized various rules and regulations intended to protect patient data security and privacy. The HIPAA regulations also extend its rules for coverage of health insurance and availability, confidentiality, and integrity of patient data. The significant features of HIPAA are listed below:

- All vital information regarding an individual's health is shared with him/her.
- The mode of exchanging health information of an individual can be chosen by them.
- The individual has the right to restrict the level of data to be exchanged with others.
- The context of patient health data exchange and purpose of sharing the data will be clearly informed to the individual.
- The individual is provided with right to consign constraint on their own health records.

HIPAA rules and regulations provide the restrictions to both doctors or healthcare practitioners and health information systems that are involved in a smart healthcare system. Doctors are provided with unambiguous guidelines for handling and sharing patient healthcare data. These guidelines also include procedures to ensure the login credentials of the individual should not be shared except with healthcare practitioners. Generally, doctors do not understand the risks involved in digital storage of data. The responsibility of ensuring the secure storage and transmission of health data will be taken care of by the information technology practitioners. The societies that are enveloped under HIPAA are known as covered entities. Wearable health monitoring devices provided by hospitals are covered under HIPAA by default. Thus, the data collected from those devices, called protected healthcare information (PHI), is completely safeguarded.

4.3.2 Federal Information Security Management Act (FISMA)

The Federal Information Security Management Act (FISMA) of 2002 is also called E-Government Act of 2002. FISMA established that the Office of Electronic Government is administrated by the Federal Chief Information Officer. The law has also mandated various sectors such as enterprise architectures of different federal agencies and security controls in IT systems that are networked nature. HIPAA rules are further strengthened by FISMA [17], which efficiently required all hospitals and healthcare providers to impose the measures to ensure the privacy and security of patients' health information. FISMA made the NIST and the Office of the Management Budget (OMB) responsible.

Based on FISMA, NIST has published two standards to confirm compliance with the act. They are Special Publications 800 series (SP-800) and Federal Information Processing Standards series (FIPS). The FIPS series provided the group of standards that federal agencies should comply with. The SP-800 series provided different constraints implied on information systems' risk profile of the organization [18, 19].

Salient features of FISMA concern the following list of actions:

- Execution of an inventory system for information systems used in the government agencies.
- Classify the information systems based on how exposed they are to risks and depict the organization's vulnerabilities to various threats.
- Identify federal systems that are extremely networked and their essential security vulnerabilities.
- As per FIPS 200, every federal organization should hold the minimal number of security controls [20].
- After classifying and allocating the minimal number of security controls, each organization has to find further information risk by performing the risk assessment. It will help to enhance the security controls for an organization.
- After completing the risk assessment security plan of the system, it will be published in accordance with the regulations of NIST.
- Once the information system is certified, then all the security controls are considered as independent functions.
- Finally, to ensure the functionalities are working properly to meet the security controls, FISMA needs a continuous monitoring system.

Table 4.1 describes a few sample laws under SP 800 and FIPS series along with their description.

FISMA 2002 was further expanded with the Cyber Enhancement Act (CEA) of 2014 [21], which concentrates on further areas of security and privacy. Some of its important features are providing a detailed guideline to do research in cyber security, maintaining the critical infrastructure for digital and physical assets of government, the significance of continuing the NIST standards, enhancing cyber security teaching in various levels such as school, college, and professional, and enhancing the awareness of cyber security.

By understanding the significant responsibility of private organizations in structure the federal information systems and also the deficient in global

Table 4.1 FISMA laws.

S. No	Law	Description of law
1	**SP800–12**	Information Security Introduction
2	**SP800–18**	Federal Information Systems security plan developing guide
3	**SP800–30**	Guide for Conducting Risk Assessments
4	**SP800–37**	Risk Management Framework for Organizations and Information Systems
5	**SP800–46**	Guide for Bring Your Own Device (BYOD) Security, Remote access and Enterprise Telework
6	**SP800–66**	Implementing the HIPAA Security Rule Resource Guide
7	**SP800–121**	Bluetooth Security Guide
8	**SP800–183**	Networks of "Things"
9	**SP800–187**	LTE Security Guide
10	**FIPS–140**	Cryptography Modules Security Requirements
11	**FIPS–199**	Information Systems and Federal Information Security Categorization Standards
12	**FIPS 200**	Information Systems and Federal Information Minimum Security necessities

consideration and interoperability made the NIST to publish the Cyber Security Framework in 2014 (CSF) [22] and further enhanced in the year 2018 [23]. In accordance with the guidelines mentioned in CSF, activities of cyber security are divided into various broad categories also called Framework Core.

4.4 Security and Privacy Issues in Smart Healthcare Based on Internet of Things

Most of IoT-based smart healthcare systems are prone to various types of security and privacy attacks.

4.4.1 Security Issues in Smart Healthcare IoT Applications

Smart healthcare includes a variety of IoT components that are exposed to various attacks. Thus, discovering and handling these security issues are among the most challenging tasks. Many researchers are still doing research in security and privacy concerns of SHC using IoT [24–27]. Confidentiality, integrity, and availability are the minimal security requirements of SHC. In this section we are going to discuss the few IoT components-based security issues such as physical objects and communication technologies.

4.4.1.1 Security Issues Related to Physical Objects

Physical objects–related security issues are listed below:

1) **Physical attacks:** IoT devices such as sensors and actuators are tiny and wirelessly connected. The data collected from sensors are health-related information, which is highly sensitive in nature so it's important to protect the stored data in IoT devices and endow the system with tools for secure storage. Since data are transmitted wirelessly, there is a high possibility of attacks and it is also easy that unauthorized data access will occur during data transmission [28]. A complete guide for IoT security is well defined by Riahi et al. [29].
2) **Amalgamate WSNs with IoT:** Wireless sensor networks integrated with IoT have restricted energy resources and battery power. WSN are generally connected all the way through loss links. This is an advantage for attackers who wish to hack the data. A malicious node deployed in the network by the attacker can damage the entire network. Securing the channel between the Internet host and the sensor node is also a challenging issue [30]. If WSN data are attacked, that will lead to life-intimidating issues of human life [31]. For acquiring the secure data storage location and availability of data there are few WSN requirements that should be considered such as data encryption and including a message authentication code.
3) **Amalgamate RFID with IoT:** Many SHC applications use RFID technology to recognize, track, and trace the patients. Because of resource constraints, RFID-based SHC systems are exposed to attacks. RFID-based IoT applications have three major components: RFID elements, middleware technology, and an Internet system [32]. These elements are exposed to many security threats such as man-in-the-middle attack, spoofing, abuse of tag, eavesdropping, and cloning. [33, 34]. To avoid peer-to-peer eavesdropping, there are symmetric and asymmetric cipher encryption in RFID systems [35].
4) **DDoS attacks:** Distributed Denial of Service (DDoS) is an attack where several malicious systems use the target system at the same time so that the system will not be available any longer. Some of the common DDoS attacks are jamming, desynchronizing attacks, kill command attacks,

and denial of sleep attack. Malicious botnet is the one of the ways to implement a DDoS attack. In recent times a newly coded malware called Mirai malware build more botnets in IoT products, which increased the total number of infected devices [36].

5) **Unauthorized access of data:** There are trillions of IoT devices available with their different users and assigned with different applications. Therefore, providing efficient authentication methods to protect the user data from the illegal access is crucial [37].

4.4.1.2 Security Issues Related to Communication Technologies

Communication technologies–related security issues are listed below:

1) **Wireless Local Area Network (WLAN) communication technologies:** WLAN communication technologies are subject to various attacks such as spying, tracking, man-in-middle attack, identifying theft disrupting network, and malicious attackers [38]. Methods to secure the data in this technology are firewalls, anti-jammers, intrusion detection, and authentication based on identity. These methods protect the data from illegal access to the network. In addition to that, encrypting schemes such as Data Encryption Standard (DES) and Advanced Encryption Standard (AES) provide the confidentiality to the data transferred in a wireless medium. Still, a physically powerful authentication is required to protect the data in communication.
2) **Wireless Wide Area Network (WWAN) communication technologies:** WWAN can be implemented using a variety of technologies. A few of them are Long Term Evolution (LTE) and Long Term Evolution-Advanced (LTE-A). LTE used to connect people from remote places using advanced technologies and low-latency traffic [39]. Generally, LTE has many security vulnerabilities such as sequence number synchronization and man-in-middle attack. To provide strong security, resistant to attacks, a new mutual authentication protocol is proposed, which is called re-authentication protocol [40]. For secure data transmission in LTE, an E-RSA (Enhanced RSA) algorithm is used. The secret key is generated using a bilinear mapping concept for a more secure key [41]. A data connection core combines the Diffie-Hellmen algorithm with a pseudorandom number generator for providing a more secure authentication scheme for a wireless environment such as LTE-A [42].
3) **IoT communication protocols:** IoT communication protocols are mapped according to the network layers as well as for a constrained-resource environment. TCP/IP layer-based communication protocols for

IoT security issues and standardized solutions are discussed in this section.

a) **Data Link Layer (DLL) communication:** DLL comprises wireless communication technologies such as LAN or WAN. In accordance with IEEE standards, IEEE 802.15.4 is the best IoT protocol because of the features such as power management and less complex modulation. This standard allows two devices to participate. They are a full-function device and a reduced-function device. Secure communication design in IEEE 802.15.4 is achieved through the MAC layer. IEEE 802.15.4 MAC layer security requirements are achieved through the AES data encryption [43], message counter to skip old messages, and verification of valid devices [44]. By using the standard 802.15.4, any message alteration in every hop can be detected, which will assure the confidentiality in the transmission route [45]. Still, it extends services such as data replay protection and data authenticity [46].
b) **Network layer communication:** When data needs to be transmitted from one end to another end over the Internet, Internet Protocol version 6 (IPv6) should be used. For ensuring the security features such as confidentiality, integrity, and authentication in data transmission in the network layer, Internet Protocol Security (IPSec) is used [45]. Along IPsec, few transport protocols can be used such as User Datagram Protocol (UDP), TCP, and HTTP. There are plenty of IoT-based IP protocols that have been proposed. Host Identity Protocol (HIP) provides better key management and secured network connection. HIP uses asymmetric key encryption, which identifies unambiguous objects and secures network connection [47]. By using a learning automata, DoS attacks can be avoided. Routing Protocol for Low Power and Lossy Networks (RPL) is a lightweight protocol, which is appropriate for constrained-resource IoT environments [48]. RPL is used in complex monitoring applications development because RPL can build the network setup fast. It also extends its support to different types of control information [49]. RPL is the fundamental protocol for 6LoWPAN (IPv6 and Low Personal Area Network) devices. They are exposed to various internal and external security attacks [50]. RPL also extends its support to confidentiality, authentication, and integrity.
c) **Transport layer communication:** UDP is the protocol that controls data packet transmission. Whenever a data packet request is received, UDP immediately initiates the packet transmission. For real-time audio- and video-related applications, UDP is the best protocol. The security protocols of transport layer are Secure Socket

Layer (SSL) and Transport Layer Security (TLS). TLS is appropriate for human interaction with web communication such as web browser and inappropriate for smart communication due to a minimal power network [51]. To overcome this disadvantage, UDP adopted Datagram Transport Layer Security (DTLS), which protects the data from DoS attacks. DTLS assured the vital features of security such as integrity, confidentiality, and authentication [52, 53]

d) **Application layer communication:** Numerous security attacks occur in the application layer such as packet loss, eavesdropping, data access in unauthorized node, and end-to-end security issues. There are many protocols available to provide secure communication in the application layer. The main ones are Message Queue Telemetry Transport (MQTT), XMPP, REST, and Constrained Application Protocol (CoAP), AMQP [54]. For constrained resources and low-cost devices, there are two famous protocols. They are MQTT and CoAP [55].

   i) **Message Queue Telemetry Transport (MQTT):** MQTT is developed by IBM. It can communicate to the multiple devices at the same time using many-to-many communication. In a wireless environment MQTT can do efficient data transmission with constrained bandwidth and energy. To connect with a client, MQTT needs a username and password. TCP connections are encrypted using SSL and TLS. To create a secure connection between server and client, TLS and SSL exploit the handshake mechanism so that an intruder cannot interpret the communication [54]. When MQTT is used with personal healthcare devices, it can combine with ISO/IEEE 11073 to minimize the data traffic [56].

   ii) **Constrained Application Protocol (CoAP):** CoAP is specifically designed for constrained-resource IoT devices. CoAP is customized for machine-to-machine (M2M) communication. It is a one-to-one communication protocol for establishing a connection between server and client for data transfer. However, maintaining security in the devices is challenging. Thus, to provide security for data transmission, DTLS is used along with UDP [43]. DTLS provides end-to-end security to the data [52, 53]. DTLS comprises three major tasks to ensure high security. They are reply detection, packet retransmission, and handshake assigning the sequence number. CoAP extends support to the sleepy devices much better than the MQTT protocol [55].

4) **Secure transmitted data:** The sensor-collected data will be transmitted through wirelessly to the remote caretakers such as doctors and nurses.

The data are vulnerable to attack while in transmission [57]. The intruders can capture and alter the patient's heath information while in transmission. Based on IBE (ID-based encryption) and PKI/CA, Yang et al. proposed a secure IoT data transmission. Secure data aggregation is another challenge in data transmission. Trust-based secure data aggregation for IoT is proposed by Liu et al. [58]. This proposed method enables secure data aggregation by using the following techniques inside of sensor nodes: data assembling and behavior identifying trust evaluation.

4.4.1.3 Security Issues Related to Applications and Cloud

Applications- and cloud storage–related security issues are listed below:

1) **Social attacks:** In this attack the intruders will disrupt human psychological factors. When a hacker wants to hack either individual or organization data, they predict the information based on their personal details such as spouse name or watching the password typing [59]. There are different types of attacks under this category. A few are listed below:
   a) **Phishing attack:** In this attack, the person may get any link or mail from a malicious source, but the user will think the mail comes from a genuine source and may open the same. As a result, a malicious user could get user credentials for accessing their details.
   b) **Baiting attack:** In this attack, the intruders will induce the people by providing some link to obtain free products. Several document-fetching software are added in this link. When the user clicks the link, the intruders can install software at the user's end.
2) **Security issues for healthcare cloud storage:** There are many security issues related to storing healthcare data in the cloud. They are:
   a) **Security issues in data access:** Health data from IoT devices are called Personal Health Records (PHR). For remote accessing of health details, PHR are stored in the cloud. PHR stored in the cloud are more vulnerable to various attacks such as man-in-middle attack and DoS/DDoS attack, which will result in false treatment to the patient, loss of health data, or modification in health data. Hence, managing the secure access of PHR in the cloud is mandatory. Still, there is a possibility of hackers modifying the health data of the patients. There are many encryption and decryption algorithms implemented for secure data access in the cloud [60]. The security algorithms include Attribute Based Encryption (ABE), Elliptic Curve Cryptography (ECC), RSA, Bilinear Maps, and Ciphertext Policy Attribute Based Encryption (CPABE). Encryption and decryption of PHR depend on healthcare service providers. For proper PHR access

at the doctor/patient end, decrypting needs the group of attributes. By combining access control and cryptographic techniques, a new cryptographic technique called Role Based Access Control technique (RBAC) has been developed to protect the PHR in the cloud. In this method, the user controls the entire data management [61].

b) **Security issues in data protection:** PHR in the cloud are stored in a shareable environment. The sensitive data about an individual patient should be maintained under a secure environment. This the biggest challenge in the cloud environment. Data encryption is one of the best solutions to secure data in cloud storage. To enhance the security of PHR from malicious cloud users, a new model is proposed called game theoretical model [62]. [63] proposes making an encrypted data backup plan to avoid the loss of PHR in cloud storage.

c) **Security issues in big data:** A collection of extremely large data having features such as volume, velocity, and variety is called big data. In healthcare, remote monitoring health information has to continuously forward from source to server. Thus, healthcare such as ECG and pulse monitoring data are big data by nature. For instance, heartbeat monitoring collected from a patient every minute may collect 4320 (72 beat × 60 minutes) data per hour, so data will be very big in size and is called big data. Moving big data into the cloud is a challenging task. Big data includes all varieties of data such as structured, semi structured, and unstructured. Structured data security can be implemented using SQL queries and existing security algorithms. Whereas unstructured data security contains four aspects of security such as hash function–based integrity, MAC is used for authenticated access control, encryption, and decryption used for confidentiality maintenance and providing authentication and identification using the signature and password verification method [64].

3) **DoS attacks on application layer:** Top layer in IoT architecture is the application layer, which comprises the user interface. One of the major issues in the application layer is DDoS/DoS attacks. DDoS/DoS attacks are classified into two major types:

a) **DDoS/DoS attacks in path:** Using an injected focus packet, an intruder creates a multi-hop end-to-end communication path. Therefore, the sensor nodes will become inundated, and the lifetime of the network also will be reduced. To avoid this attack, defense methods such as packet authentication and anti-reply protection are used [65].

b) **Reprogramming attack:** An intruder is capable of getting entire access (modify/control) to the source code, which will end up with numerous application request to the network sources. To avoid this attack, an authentication stream can be implemented [66].

4) **Attacks on web application:** There are many attacks associated with the healthcare applications such as SQL injection attacks, cross-site request forgery attack (CSRF), and XSS (cross-site scripting) attack.
   a) **SQL injection attack:** In this attack, an intruder attempts to inject the SQL query from the user to the application. Therefore, the intruder can control the database management system. Database administration operations are also controlled by an SQL injection attack. SQL injection attacks result in integrity, authentication, authorization, and confidentiality issues [67].
   b) **Cross-site request forgery attack (CSRF):** This is also called one-click or session-riding attack. In this attack, a malicious user request is transmitted to a website without the consent of authorized access persons of that website [68]. The website cannot differentiate whether the requests came from an authenticated user or not. CSRF attacks can be avoided by using website protection mechanisms or personal protection mechanisms [69]. CSRF guard is a tool that runs on the Java Enterprise Edition environment to defend against CSRF attacks [70].

4.4.2 Privacy Issues in Smart Healthcare IoT Applications

The privacy issues involved in IoT-based smart healthcare applications along with their solutions are discussed in the following section.

1) Patient Privacy Exposure Risk
   PHR can gather information from various sources for sharing, managing, and controlling the health data by an individual person [71]. The most important issue in PHR is keeping the patient information confidential. Before sharing, the PHR encryption algorithms are applied to encrypt the PHR data. Algorithms such as AES and Message Digest 5 (MD5) are combined with efficient key management to encrypt the files in PHR [72].
2) Cyberattack Threats on Privacy
   In a cyberattack, false information can be infused into the system, which causes heavy damage to the IoT healthcare applications. Therefore, it is mandatory to give sufficient protection to the healthcare applications against cyberattacks. Still, because of the resource-constrained IoT environment, security implementations against cyberattacks are challenging. By considering the decision cost minimization approach, a novel

distributed cyberattack detection algorithm is proposed [73]. This method detects the unknown and known cyberattacks efficiently. Tajer et al. designed a framework that is used to detect cyberattacks and recover from the same. To detect cyberattacks constituted the following subsystems, different controlling agents along distributed across the network [74].

4.5 Issues in Location Privacy

Location privacy is included with location-related issues such as eavesdropping and DoS. Location privacy in a sensor can be achieved by routing through a randomly chosen intermediate node to hide the data sender's location [75]. By using the Location Privacy Routing (LPR) protocol, tracing of data packets and eavesdropping can be avoided [76]. This method is based on the direction of incoming and outgoing traffic at individual sensor nodes, which are uniformly distributed.

4.6 Issues in Privacy of Stored Data and Threats Identity

Patient privacy includes many attributes such as confidentiality and identity. When patients face issues where their identity or confidential information is revealed, this leads to many harmful situations physically, emotionally, and sometimes also financially. Hence, Slamanig et al. proposed mechanisms to avoid the disclosure attacks using features such as unlinkability, anonymity, pseudonymity, and identity management. Pseudonymity and anonymity are used to hide the identity that is connected with the stored data. To protect the health records, differential privacy techniques are used along merging a noise to a patient's health data, which results in assuring privacy in PHR [77].

4.7 Conclusion

The modern growth in IoT results in advanced solutions to various areas such as smart agriculture, smart inventory systems, and smart healthcare systems. Maintaining the security of data is nowadays crucial. Thus, protecting the security and privacy of the data at all stages of data flow is among the most important research areas. Still, there are plenty of issues and challenges in security and privacy of IoT-based smart healthcare systems. In this chapter we discussed the overview of smart healthcare architecture, rules and regulations involved in implementation of smart healthcare applications, and security and privacy issues with some of the existing solutions in detail. The technical specifications and standards are still improving specifically in the requirements of healthcare applications, so a detailed examination is still needed.

Author Biography

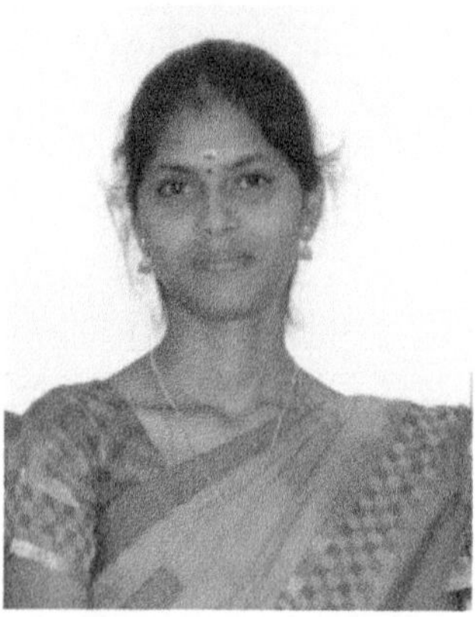

Dr. R. Nidhya is presently working as associate professor in the Department of Computer Science & Engineering, Madanapalle Institute of Technology & Science, affiliated to Jawaharlal Nehru Technical University, Anantapuram, India. She received the M. Tech and PhD degrees from Anna University, Chennai. Her research interests include wireless body area networks, network security, and machine learning. She has published many research papers in refereed international journals and IEEE and Springer associated conferences. She is an active member of professional societies such as CSI, ISTE, SAISE, and ISRD.

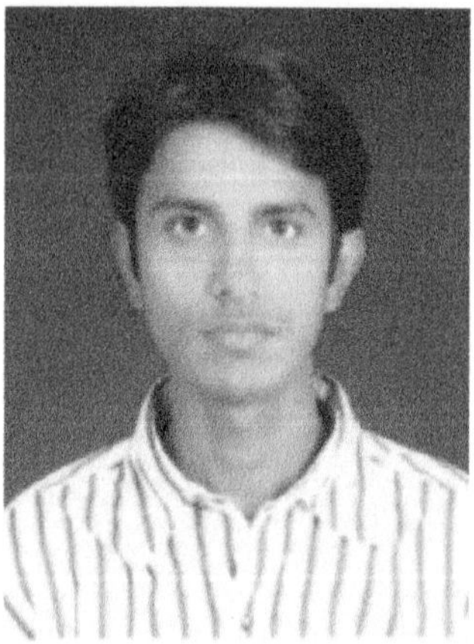

Dr. Manish Kumar received his B.E. degree in information technology from Rajiv Gandhi Technical University, Bhopal, India, in 2011 and a PhD degree from Indian Institute of Technology (Indian School of Mines), Dhanbad, in 2018. He is currently working as an assistant professor in the School of Computer Science & Engineering, VIT, Chennai. His research interests include soft computing applications for bioinformatics problems and computational intelligence.

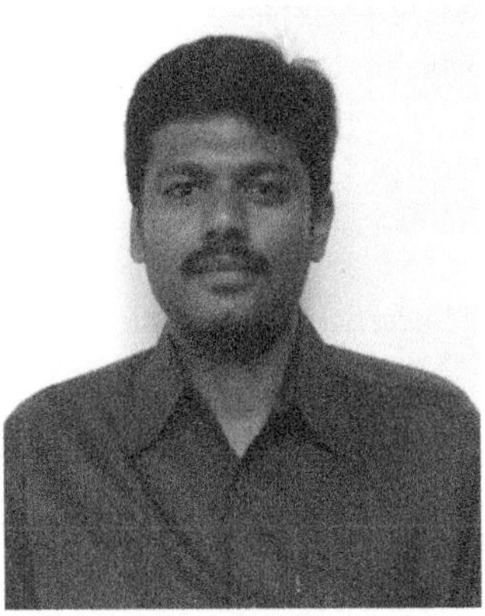

R. Maheswar has completed his B.E. (ECE) from Madras University in 1999, M.E. (Applied Electronics) from Bharathiyar University in 2002, and PhD in the field of wireless sensor networks from Anna University in 2012. He has about 15 years of teaching experience at various levels and is presently working as a professor in the Electronics and Communication Engineering Department, Sri Krishna College of Technology, Coimbatore, Tamil Nadu, India. He has published 40 papers at international journals and international conferences. His research interests include wireless sensor networks, queueing theory, and performance evaluation.

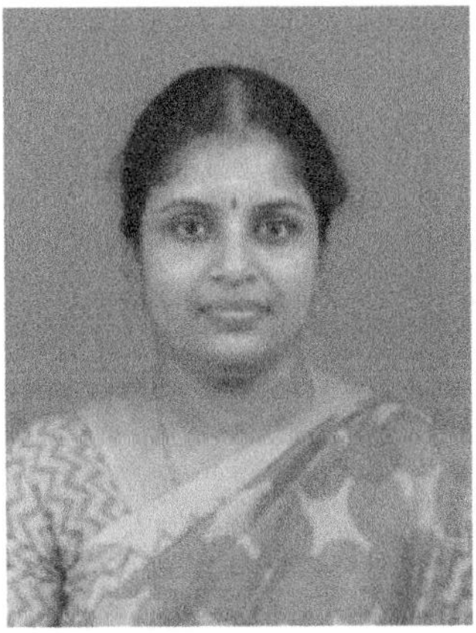

D. Pavithra is currently a research scholar in the Department of Electronics and Communication Engineering, Sri Ramakrishna Institute of Technology, Coimbatore, Tamil Nadu, India. She received a bachelor's degree B.E. (computer hardware and software engineering) from Avinashilingam Deemed University, Coimbatore in 2002. Then she completed her M.E. (computer science) in Dr. Mahalingam College of Engineering and Technology, Pollachi, under Anna Unniversity, Coimbatore, in 2011. Her current research interests include autism, machine learning, and deep learning.

References

1 Nidhya, R. and Karthik, S. (2019). Security and privacy issues in remote healthcare systems using wireless body area networks. In: *Body Area Network Challenges and Solutions* (eds. R. Maheswar, G. Kanagachidambaresan, R. Jayaparvathy and S. Thampi). EAI/Springer Innovations in Communication and Computing.

2 Hussain, A., Wenbi, R., da Silva, A.L. et al. (2015). Health and emergency-care platform for the elderly and disabled people in the Smart City. *Journal of Systems and Software* 110: 253–263.

3 Li, J., Liu, Z., Chen, X. et al. (2015). LEncDB: a lightweight framework for privacy-preserving data queries in cloud computing. *Knowledge-Based Systems* 79: 18–26.

4 Lin, Q., Li, J., Huang, Z. et al. (2018). A short linearly homomorphic proxy signature scheme. *IEEE Access* 6: 12966–12972.

5 Xie, R., He, C., Xie, D. et al. A secure ciphertext retrieval scheme against insider KGAs for mobile devices in cloud storage. *Security and Communication Networks* 2018: DOI:https://doi.org/10.1155/2018/7254305.

6 Zhang, Y., Li, J., Chen, X., and Li, H. (2016). Anonymous attribute-based proxy re-encryption for access control in cloud computing. *Security and Communication Networks* 9 (14): 2397–2411.

7 Yuan, C., Li, X., Wu, Q.J. et al. (2015). Fingerprint liveness detection from different fingerprint materials using convolutional neural network and principal component analysis. *Computers, Materials & Continua* 53 (4): 357–371.

8 Li, J., Chen, X., Chow, S.S.M. et al. (2018). Multi-authority fine-grained access control with accountability and its application in cloud. *Journal of Network and Computer Applications.*

9 Zhang, Y., Zheng, D., and Deng, R.H. (2018). Security and privacy in smart health: efficient policy-hiding attribute-based access control. *IEEE Internet of Things Journal* 5 (3): 2130–2145.

10 Li, P., Li, J., and Huang, Z. (2017). Multi-key privacy-preserving deep learning in cloud computing. *Future Generation Computer Systems* 74: 76–85.

11 Zhang, Y., Chen, X., Li, J. et al. (2013). Anonymous attribute-based encryption supporting efficient decryption test. In: *Proceedings of the 8th ACMSIGSAC Symposium on Information, Computer and Communications Security*, 511–516. ACM.

12 Li, J., Chen, X., Li, M. et al. (2014). Secure deduplication with efficient and reliable convergent key management. *IEEE Transactions on Parallel and Distributed Systems* 25 (6): 1615–1625.

13 Li, P., Li, J., Huang, Z. et al. (2017). Privacy-preserving outsourced classification in cloud computing. *Cluster Computing* (1): 1–10.

14 Nidhya, R., Arunchalam, V.P., and Karthick, S. (2016). Multitier security architecture with energy requirement for medical wireless sensor network. *International Journal of Printing, Packaging & Allied Sciences* 4 (5).

15 www.nist.gov

16 https://www.gpo.gov/fdsys/pkg/BILLS-104s1028is/pdf/BILLS-104s1028is.pdf

17 https://csrc.nist.gov/topics/laws-and-regulations/laws/fisma

18 https://csrc.nist.gov/publications/fips
19 https://csrc.nist.gov/publications/sp800
20 https://www.nist.gov/publications/minimum-security-requirements-federal-information-and-information-systems-federal
21 https://www.gpo.gov/fdsys/pkg/PLAW-113publ283/pdf/PLAW-113publ283.pdf
22 https://www.nist.gov/cyberframework/framework-version-10
23 https://www.nist.gov/cyberframework/new-framework
24 Aggarwal, C.C. and Yu, P.S. (2008). *An Introduction to Privacy- Preserving Data Mining, Privacy-Preserving data Mining Models and Algorithms*, 1e, 1–9. New York: Springer US.
25 Weber, R.H. (2010). Internet of things - new security and privacy challenges. *Computer Law & Security Report* 26 (1): 23–30.
26 Sue, H., Wan, J., Zou, C., and Liu, J. (2012). Security in the internet of things: a review. In: *IEEE International Conference on Computer Science and Electronics Engineering*, vol. 3, 648–651.
27 Matharu, G.S., Upadhyay, P., and Chaudhary, L. (2014). The internet of things: challenges and security issues. In: *IEEE International Conference on Emerging Technologies*, Islamabad, 54–59.
28 Gambs et al. (2014). Nov. 19, 2014. IoT privacy, data protection, information security. Available on: http://licit.inrialpes.fr/apvp2010/slides/apvp_adept_gambs.pdf.
29 Riahi, A., Challal, Y., Natalizio, E. et al. (2013). A systemic approach for IoT security. In: *IEEE International Conference on Distributed Computing in Sensor Systems*, Boston, 351–355.
30 Tharani, M. (2014). Integrating wireless sensor networks into internet of things for security. *International Journal of Advanced Research In Computer Science and Management Studies* 1 (2): 485–490.
31 Mainetti, L., Patrono, L., and Vilei, A. (2011). Evaluation of wireless sensor networks towards the internet of things: a survey. In: *IEEE 19th International Conference on Software, Telecommunications and Computer Networks*, 1–6.
32 Nie, X. and Zhong, X. (2013). Security the internet of things based on RFID: issues and current countermeasures. In: *Proceedings of the 2nd International Conference on Computer Science and Electronics Engineering*, 1181–1184.
33 Khoo, B. (2011). RFID as a enabler of the internet of things: issues of security and privacy. In: *IEEE 4th International Conference on Cyber, Physical and Social Computing*, 709–712.
34 Jia, X., Feng, Q., Fan, T., and Lei, Q. (2012). RFID technology and its applications in internet of things (IOT). In: *IEEE 2nd International Conference on Consumer Electronics, Communications and Networks*, 1282–1285.

35 Finkenzeller, K. (2009). Known attacks on RFID systems, possible countermeasures and upcoming standardization activities. In: *5th European Workshop on RFID Systems and Technologies*, 1–31.

36 K. Michael, Hackers create more IoT botnets with Mirai source code," PCWorld, http://www.pcworld.com/article/3132571/hackerscreate-more-iot-botnets-with-mirai-source-code.html, 2006.

37 Sain, M., Kumar, P., and Lee, H.J. (2011). Secure authentication and communication in ubiquitous healthcare middleware. In: *IEEE 13th International Conference, Advanced Communication Technology*, 173–178.

38 Choi, M.K., Robles, R.J., Hong, C.H., and Kim, T.H. (2008). Wireless network security: vulnerabilities, threats and countermeasures. *International Journal of Multimedia and Ubiquitous Engineering* 3: 77–86.

39 M2M Connectivity. Available on:, Last access June 16, 2015. http://blog.m2mconnectivity.com.au/category/internet-of-things.

40 Bouabidi, I.E., Daly, I., and Zarai, F. (2012). Secure handoff protocol in 3GPP LTE networks. In: *IEEE 3rd International Conference on Communications and Networking*, 1–6.

41 Nidhya, R., Shanthi, S., and Kumar, M. (2021). A novel encryption design for wireless body area network in remote healthcare system using enhanced RSA algorithm. In: *Intelligent System Design*, Advances in Intelligent Systems and Computing, vol. 1171 (eds. S. Satapathy, V. Bhateja, B. Janakiramaiah and Y.W. Chen).

42 Huang, Y.L., Leu, F.Y., Liu, J.C. et al. (2013). A secure wireless communication system integration PRNG and Diffie-Hellman PKDS by using a data connection core. In: *IEEE 8th International Conference on Wireless Computing, Communication and Applications*, 360–365.

43 Granjal, J., Monteiro, E., and Silva, J. (2015). Security of the internet of things: a survey of existing protocols and open research issues. *IEEE Communication Surveys and Tutorials*: 1.

44 Xiao, Y., Sethi, S., Chen, H.H., and Sun, B. (2005). Security services and enhancements in the IEEE 802.15.4 wireless sensor networks. *IEEE Global Communications Conference* 3: 1796–1800.

45 Raza, S., Duquennoy, S., Chung, T. et al. (2011). Securing communication in 6LoWPAN with compressed IPsec. In: *IEEE International Conference on Distributed Computing in Sensor Systems and Workshops*, 1–8.

46 Daidone, R., Dini, G., and Tiloca, M. (2011). On experimentally evaluating the impact of security on IEEE 802.15.4 networks. In: *IEEE International Conference on Distributed Computing in Sensor Systems and Workshops*, 1–6.

47 Meca, F.V. and Ziegeladorf, J.H. (2013). HIP security architecture for the IP-based internet of things. In: *IEEE 27th International Conference on Advanced Information Networking and Applications Workshops*, 1331–1336.

48 Pongle, P. and Chavan, G. (2015). A survey: attacks on RPL and 6LoWPAN in IoT. In: *IEEE International Conference on Pervasive Computing*, 1–6.

49 Accettura, N., Grieco, L.A., Boggia, G., and Camarda, P. (2011). Peformance analysis of the RPL routing protocol. In: *IEEE International Conference on Mechatronics*, 767–772.

50 Le, A., Loo, J., Luo, Y., and Lasebae, A. (2011). Specification-based IDS for securing RPL from toplogy attacks. In: *IEEE IFIP Wireless Days*, 1–3.

51 Designing the Internet of Things, Available on: http://micrium.com/iot/internet-protocols,. Last access June 16, 2015

52 Nidhya, R., Karthik, S., and Smilarubavathy, G. (2019). An end-to-end secure and energy-aware routing mechanism for IoT-based modern health care system. In: *Soft Computing and Signal Processing*, Advances in Intelligent Systems and Computing, vol. 900 (eds. J. Wang, G. Reddy, V. Prasad and V. Reddy).

53 E. Rescorla and N. Modadugu, Datagram Transport Layer Security Version 1.2, RFC6347, 2012. Available on: http://www.ietf.org/rfc6347.txt, Last access June 1, 2015.

54 Karagiannis, V., Chatzimisios, P., Gallego, F.V., and Zarate, J.A. (2015). A survey on application layer protocols for the internet of things. In: *Transactions on IoT and Cloud Computing*, 1–10.

55 Collina, M., Bartolucci, M., Coralli, A.V., and Corazza, G.E. (2014). Internet of things application layer protocol analysis over error and delay prone links. In: *IEEE Advanced Satellite Multimedia System Conference and the 13th Signal Processing for Space Communications Workshop*, 398–404.

56 Gomes, Y.F., Santos, D.F.S., Almeida, H.O., and Perkusich, A. (2015). Integrating MQTT and IS/IEEE 11073 for health information sharing in the internet of things. In: *IEEE International Conference on Consumer Electronics*, 200–201.

57 H-Ramos, J.L., Bernabé, J.B., and Skarmeta, A.F. (2014). Towards privacy-preserving data sharing in smart environments. In: *IEEE 8th International Conference on Innovative Mobile and Internet Services in Ubiquitous Computing*, 334–339.

58 Liu, Y., Gong, X., and Xing, C. (2014). A novel trust-based secure data aggregation for internet of things. In: *IEEE 9th International Conference on Computer Science and Education*, 435–439.

59 https://www.tripwire.com/state-of-security/security-awareness/5-social-engineering-attacks-to-watch-out-for

60 Alshehri, S., Radziszowski, S.P., and Raj, R.K. (2012). Secure access foe healthcare data in the cloud using Ciphertext-policy attribute-based encryption. In: *IEEE 28th International Conference on Data Engineering Workshops*, 143–146.

61 Zhou, L., Varadharajan, V., and Hitchens, M. (2013). Integrating trust with cryptographic role- based access control for secure data storage. In: *IEEE 12th International Conference on Trust, Security and Privacy in Computing and Communications*, 560–569.

62 Jebalia, M., Letaifa, A.B., Hamdi, M., and Tabbane, S. (2014). A revocation game model for secure cloud storage. In: *IEEE International Conference on High Performance Computing and Simulation*, 1016–1017.

63 Mxoli, A., Gerber, M., and Phipps, N.M. (2014). Information security risk measures for cloud-based personal heath records. In: *IEEE International Conference on Information Society*, 187–193.

64 Islam, M.R. and Islam, M.E. (2014). An approach to provide security to unstructured big data. In: *IEEE International Conference on Software, Knowledge, Information Management and Applications*, 1–5.

65 Yu, C.M., Tsou, Y.T., Lu, C.S., and Kuo, S.Y. (2011). Constrained function-based message authentication for sensor networks. *IEEE Transactions on Information Forensics and Security* 6: 407–425.

66 Li, Q. and Trappe, W. (2006). Reducing delay and enhancing DoS resistance in multicast authentication through multigame security. *IEEE Transactions on Information Forensics and Security* 1: 190–204.

67 Yan, Y., Zhengyuan, S., and Zucheng, D. (2011). The database protection system against SQL attacks. In: *IEEE 3rd International Conference on Computer Research and Development*, vol. 3, 99–102.

68 Siddiqui, M.S. and Verma, D. (2011). Cross site request forgery: a common web application weakness. In: *IEEE 3rd International Conference on Communication Software and Networks*, Xi'an, 538–543.

69 J. Blatz, CSRF: Attack and Defense, Available on: http://www.mcafee.com/us/resources/white-papers/wp-csrf-attack-defense.pdf,Last access June 7, 2015.

70 You, J. and Guo, F. (2014). Improved CSRF guard for CSRF attacks defense on Java EE platform. In: *IEEE 9th International Conference on Computer Science and Education*, 1115–1120.

71 Khan, J.S., Aulakh, V., and Bosworth, A. What it takes: characteristics of the ideal personal health record. *Health Affairs (Millwood)* 28 (2): 369–376.

72 Manda, S.K. and Hanmanthu, B. (2013). Privacy preserving support for mobile health care using message digest. *International Journal of Advanced Research in Computer Science and Software Engineering* 3: 197–102.

73 Nguyen, H.D., Gutta, S., and Cheng, Q. (2010). An active distributed approach for cyber attack detection. In: *IEEE Conference on Signals, Systems and Computers*, 1540–1544.

74 Tajer, A., Kar, S., Poor, H.V., and Cui, S. (2011). Distributed joint cyber attack detection and state recovery in smart grids. In: *IEEE International Conference on Smart Grid Communications*, 202–207.

75 Ren, J., Li, Y., and Li, T. (2009). Routing-based source-location privacy in wireless sensor networks. In: *IEEE International Conference on Communications*, 1–5.

76 Jian, Y., Chen, S., Zhang, Z., and Zhang, L. (2007). Protecting receiver-location privacy in wireless sensor networks. In: *IEEE 26th International Conference on Computer Communications*, 1955–1963.

77 Hall, R., Rinaldo, A., and Wasserman, L. (2013). Differential privacy for functions and functional data. *Journal of Machine Learning Research*: 703–727.

5

An Overview of Architecture and Applications of IoT-Based Health Care Systems

M. Saravanan[1], J. Ajayan[2], R. Maheswar[3], and E. Parthasarathy[4]

[1] *Department of Electronics and Communication Engineering, Sri Eshwar College of Engineering, Coimbatore, Tamilnadu, India*
[2] *Department of Electronics and Communication Engineering, SR University, Warangal, Telangana, India*
[3] *School of Electrical & Electronics Engineering (SEEE), VIT Bhopal University, Sehore, Madhya Pradesh, India*
[4] *Department of Electronics and Communication Engineering, SRM Institute of Science and Technology, Chennai, Tamilnadu, India*

5.1 Introduction

In our modern world, technology has been improving substantially; it affects most, if not all, of our society, and the healthcare system is not an exception. Healthcare systems in certain countries have improved substantially to provide better treatment for their people; these countries provide better treatment because of monitoring their patients' conditions consistently, helping them to recover from their diseases.

For example, people who suffer from diabetes need a doctor's advice regularly; diabetes causes abnormal function of the pancreas. This leads to vital organ damage. By using the applications of IoT, the sensors embedded with the system that continuously sense and monitor the patients' health and send the recorded data to their doctors can reduce the risk of death.

IoT in healthcare services has received growing attention due to the rapid technological advancement of sensor devices, sensor networks, and mobile data transmission. It can collect, store, record, and analyze the data, which can be further streamed with much faster speed [1].

IoT-Enabled Smart Healthcare Systems, Services and Applications, First Edition.
Edited by Shalli Rani, Maheswar Rajagopal, Neeraj Kumar and Syed Hassan Ahmed Shah.

The miniaturization of sensors helps to reduce the material cost as well as power consumption. It focuses much on the increase in quality care. These provide a better solution for measurement of various body parameters such as ECG (Electrocardiography), temperature, moisture, and heartbeat. The performance of these sensors can be evaluated based on specific vital parameters such as sensitivity, linearity, selectivity, the limit of detection, dynamic range, the precision of the response, reproducibility, response to interferences, portability, ease of use, operational stability, and response time [10]. Biosensors constitute a multidisciplinary field that has recently emerged as a vital area of research.

An important benefit of the system is its portability; it is remotely connected to the cloud, so it can be carried anywhere without any disturbances. Additional benefits are that tracking and monitoring can be done in real time, the measured parameters are also accurate, it is a completely automated workflow, so there is no wastage of time, and it will cut down medical costs by half, as there is no need to visit hospitals regularly.

5.2 Overview of the Healthcare System

In IoT based health care system, sensors are connected with our body which used to measure various body parameters, these sensors are connected with a microcontroller which will send measured parameters to data control center where data will get processed, the micro-controller selection is based upon the various usage and portability purposes, such as Arduino, Raspberry Pi. Pi. It collects the data from the sensor and transmits them for further level (Figure 5.1).

Then, a microcontroller sends the data to a cloud database; Data collected in the IoT are stored in a relational database system, so it can be used for analytical purpose and also for user who are connected with their smartphones can able to view their health status in their past days [2]. Around the globe, there are different cloud-based organizations. Their purpose is not only to provide the best storage but also to improve user security over the data. The server is where they used to get the data and also fetch the data [13]; here the user can also calculate their health parameters for their health-related issues. If the patient is under a critical situation, it also sends the data to the emergency services such as doctors or EMTs and to close relatives [4]. From this, it can be detected whether the patient needs medical assistance.

In this chapter, we are going to describe the various existing sensors as well as their working principles and the emerging sensors that are being currently developed.

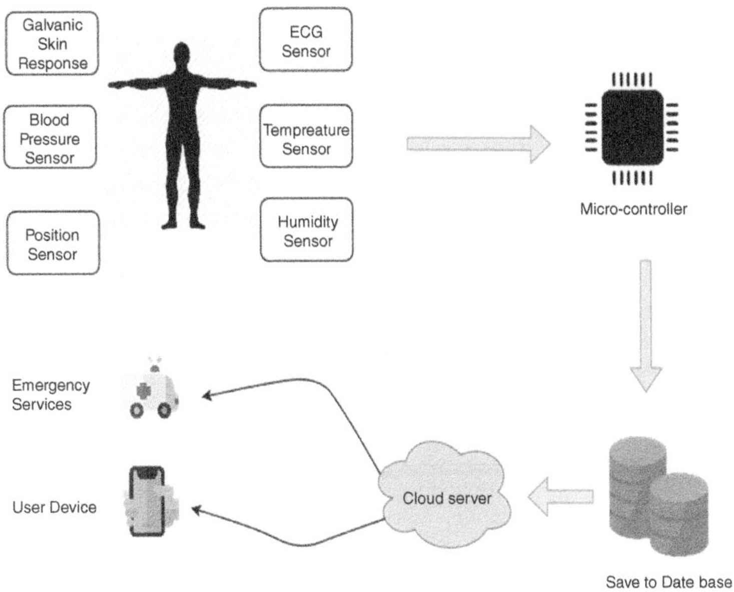

Figure 5.1 Architecture of health care system.

5.3 Working Prototype of Healthcare System Using BAN

In first stage, data is collected from user such as patient so this stage is called as collection phase. The data collected may vary for different diseases. Similarly, Devices that measure various parameters are connected through IoT. The devices connected in the patient's body are called body area network; this system collects data, which is then transmitted to a server. In the transmission phase, the microcontroller plays the main role, processing the received signals, i.e., the sensor responses from the BAN (body area network) [18]. A GSM module is mounted together with the Raspberry Pi, and it has complete access to sending and receiving the data form the patient; this can be controlled by the standard AT commands The GSM module paves the way to communicate between the cloud server and the user; the data transfer is quite fast making it reliable. A database connection is also provided for research purposes and to allow the doctor to track the patient's records. It provides two-way communication, transmitting and receiving the data. Micro controller are programmed with critical level of that disease, such as blood pressure, when a person reach low blood pressure that range is already programmed. [18–20]. It alerts the doctor as well as a patient's relative.

The detailed flow of the system architecture is explained in Figure 5.2, When the patient is in need of medical help, the microcontroller sends the signal to the cloud server; the measured parameter is in analog form, and for data processing, it needs to be converted into digital form [23] via the GSM module to the database system, which responds to the data and sends the alert to the doctor and the medical emergency services. If the collected data is not in the range of critical values, the information is only stored in the cloud without any notification. The complete process is done on this IOT-based service.

5.3.1 Microcontroller (Raspberry Pi)

Raspberry Pi is a type of microcontroller used for automating a process; many industries are using it as their main component. Raspberry Pi is also used as an information collector in addition to a processor. Its board provides a set of pins, named general-purpose input and output pins, which allow it to control electronic components for physical computing, and therefore, it is widely applicable in the IoT (Figure 5.3).

The processor used in the proposed method is a 3rd generation processor, it is 10 times faster than the first generation, and it has wireless local area

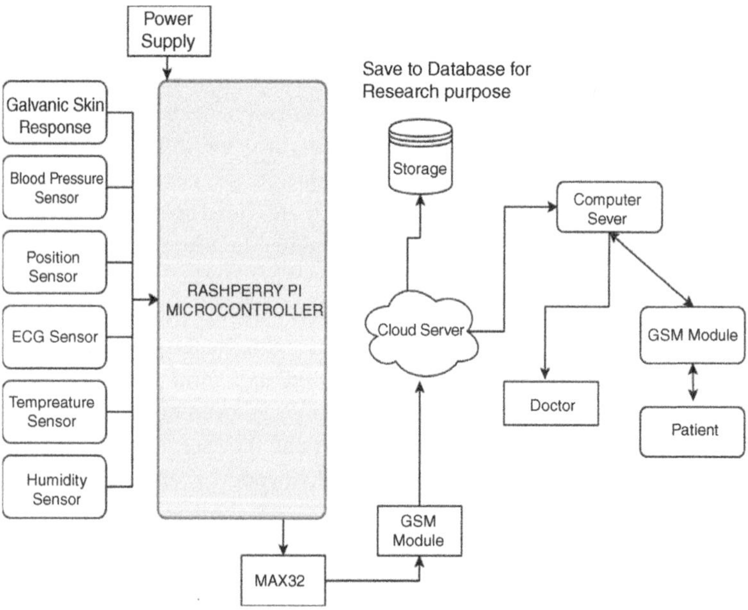

Figure 5.2 Working flow of health care system.

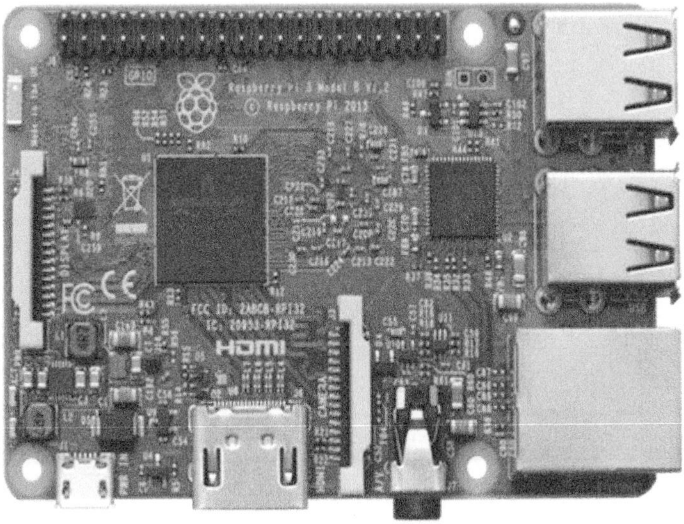

Figure 5.3 Raspberry Pi module.

network (LAN) and Bluetooth options [22]. The GPIO (General Purpose Input/Output) connector has 40 pins by configuration (20×2), pin 27 acts as +3.3V, +5V, and the GND supplies lines [3–21]. It improves added connectivity and lower cost.

The board uses the Debian operating system. This OS is highly optimized for the Pi microprocessor and is also lightweight. Compared to their previous version, the Pi 3, it has single-threaded performance, which is greatly improved; its biggest advantage is that it is possible to gain multi-threaded programs. A minimum size of a 2GB SD card is required to preinstall the Raspbian OS, but a 4GB SD card or above is highly recommended for future addition of packages.

5.3.2 Adopting Wearables and IOT

Wearable devices are the heart of the technological world. With technological development, doctors are able to remotely access all health parameters of patients; nowadays healthcare devices act as personal doctors by virtual visits; they measure body parameters for us, such as the fitness tracker, which consistently monitors the calories burned in our body and tracks the distance traveled, and so on. Wearable gadgets have the functionality to improve their communication, for which IoT helps them. Some functionalities of the gadgets are related to identification and security in work

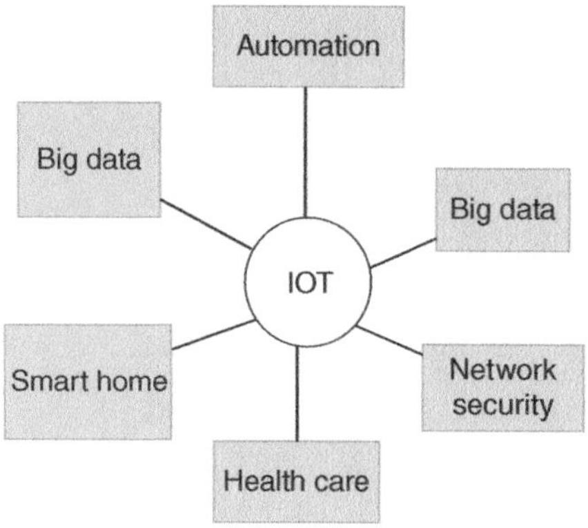

Figure 5.4 Integrating IOT ecosystem.

environments. The more reliable devices provide the accurate location of the patient [10]. A better model allows each device to connect to all surrounding devices. Internet of Things promises to handle large number of collections without any data loss and also data transferring are highly interactable with larger infrastructure. (Figure 5.4).

The architecture associated with the wearable gadgets has many levels of integration techniques to the user interface. A similar example is the Bluetooth connected to the patient's smartphone, which is a very popular method to transfer information, but it is not used for all purposes [24]. For research purposes, a sports player's entire stats can be viewed by their coach and his medical staff; this shows the live feature of observing the data sending acknowledgment to the cloud servers.

5.3.3 Wearable Backend Servers

The physical mechanisms are in the collection phase, including collecting data from the electronic devices, and then the transmission to backend servers begin to take part in processing and storing the data. The cloud storage providers take care of handling and managing the data fed into their servers; Amazon Web Services, SAP, and Microsoft Azure are the leading firms. To provide flexible operations over the data, software networking can be used to customize the data collection separately. These backend servers acts as bridge in the human-cloud integration [24]. It also requires the hardware support system to achieve complete functionality. By analyzing the cloud data, it provides real-time solutions for the medical healthcare systems for users' health statuses. For example, if a user BP went below the normal range, the server sends the information to the necessary medical emergency personnel.

5.4 On-Body Sensors and Sensor Embodiment

According to the report of WHO (World Health Organization) in last decade diabetes caused 1.5 million deaths; to reduce these kinds of health-related risks, on-body sensors are used for monitoring the health status regularly. The BSN (ody sensor network) hardware has incorporated various sensor such as smart sensors and bio-chemical sensors. The hardware is mainly focused on the wireless communication and low-power processing of the signals [1].

5.4.1 Smart Sensors

Smart sensors are devices that can perform more than one logical function, such as a two-way communication mechanism, which makes their own decision. Sensors use a property of transduction of class materials and their electronic properties. These transduction elements are included with thin metal films, zinc oxide, or polymeric films. Electronic components integrated with these ICs provide an easier solution. Flexible electronics have an increasing role in health screening and treatment processes. The smart sensors can also be coupled with nanotechnology and smartphones, providing an improved result in data analysis [25]. This is widely used for detection of various types of diseases and for healthcare monitoring. There are several multidisciplinary organizations developing smart sensors.

The building blocks of the smart sensors are sensing units and communication units. Initially the signals condition is tested and converted from analog to digital; the application algorithm of the smart sensors is integrated with the memory unit for programmatic needs. Later on the signal is driven to the transceiver unit. It can also have an advantage over other alternatives: it calibrates sensors in batch processes during the production environment or test fixture. The following are the main uses of smart sensors:

- Due to an increased visibility of the IoT, smart sensors enable real-data control. For example, in some logistic companies transportation has an important role, and fleet vehicles can be tracked by these devices.
- By making use of smart sensors, lots of cables and connectors can be eliminated.
- Very weak electrical signals are produced as an output in other sensors,. This mainly avoids weak signals transmitting over the cables.

Smart sensors currently have the ability to calculate more than one variable simultaneously, such as physical or chemical. In smart sensors, it is possible to make simple checks that arise during the transmission time as a common fault; they are all self-diagnosed. Some of them are storing different values in memory unit because of calculating the minimum and maximum in the device itself. This makes data completely usable if any data is interrupted as false. Even though smart sensors can be integrated in a single silicon chip, they are expensive. A silicon chip can do both analog and digital processing and can also have non-volatile memory (NVRAM).

5.4.2 Gas Sensors

There are certain gases thatare more prone to human bodies such as carbon monoxide (CO), which is an odorless and tasteless gas; when CO enters the human body at certain concentration, it will negatively affect and could even kill the person [27], so providing a gas sensor will reduce the risk. These sensors measure the concentration of a particular gas in the atmosphere. Sensors produce a measurable amount of electrical current when chemical reactions caused by the specific gas take place. The sensor monitors these currents and warns the patient when a certain amount of a dangerous gas reaches a threshold. The main component of a gas sensor is the gas-sensing layer, which senses the gases of various concentrations and then produces a change in electrical resistance (Table 5.1). An example is chemiresister, which is made of tin dioxide (SnO2). This is how it works: in clean air there are no free electrons present, so there is no current produced, but when there are toxic gases, the level of oxygen is lower, which means fewer combustible gases are present; this causes a free flow of electrons and current. [26].

Gas sensors have the following main components: (Figure 5.5):

- **Sensing layer:** Its aim is to detect the presence of various gases in the atmosphere.
- **Electrode line:** The result of the sensing layer is fed into the electrode line where these are connected by the junction; it produces a small amount of current and helps in moving the electrons efficiently.

Table 5.1 Comparison table of gas sensors and its concepts.

Type of sensor	Advantage	Disadvantage
Metal oxide sensor	Low cost, wide range of gases are sensed, little maintenance, good for miniaturization.	Large power consumption, requires oxygen, major dependencies on ambient temperature and humidity.
Electrochemical sensor	Low cost, broad target of gases is sensed, ultra-low power consumption.	Slow response time, high maintenance on using electrolytes.

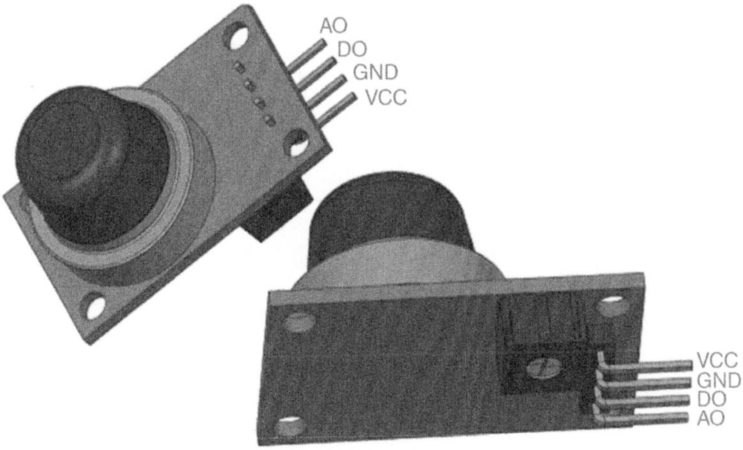

Figure 5.5 Schematic diagram of gas sensor.

5.4.3 Bio-Chemical Sensors

The biochemical sensor improves the detection limits and selectivity for the qualification of biological analytes. These sensors are used in medical diagnosis, monitoring the environment, clinical chemistry, agriculture, and military detection to detect chemical and biological warfare agents.

Bio-chemical sensors are analytical devices that convert a biological response into an electrical signal and then monitor the electrolyte concentration and pH in the sweat and are even able to detect specific components. The transducer in bio-chemical sensors is made up of an ISFET (ion-sensitive field-effect transistor) or a chemFET (chemically sensitive field-effect transistor). An enzyme biosensor uses immobilized biocatalysts such as a single or multiple enzymes, which recognize, bind, and subsequently transform the target analytes (substrates). In enzymatic sensors, both the enzyme inhibition and catalytic conversion of the substrate can be used to monitor the analyte [27].

A biosensor has three segments: a sensor, transducers, and electrons associated with it (Figure 5.6). Modern biochemical sensors are based on the micro-reactor construction. The basic characteristics of sensors are linearity, higher concentration of substrate, and sensitivity of the bio-sensor electrode [28–30]. These sensors are characterized by having response time of about 33 s and an operational stability over 3 weeks. And the chemicals interference is minimized in obtaining the result. Its advantages are relatively a long life, an acceptable price range, and accurate results.

The sensors have four components: analyte, bioreceptor, transducer, and detector. In the analyte section the signals are received and then transferred

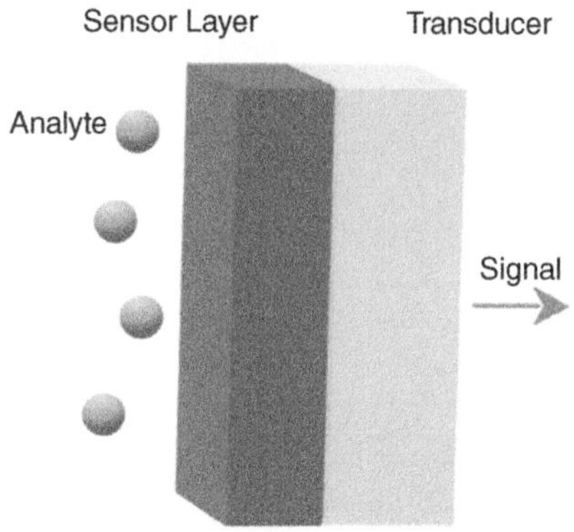

Figure 5.6 Segments of biochemical sensor.

to the bioreceptors; these signals are the enzymes and antibody and microorganisms. Similarly to the smart sensors, the biochemical sensors also carry out real-time diagnosis of various diseases. Environmental studies involve many steps such as sample handling and sample transportation.

The biosensors are regenerated by replacing the enzymatic membrane with another one. Replacement processes may be difficult sometimes, so the modular system approach is carried out. Nanotechnology is an emerging field in all chemical-based sectors. It enables to fabricate functional materials and to exploit their properties. The fabricated sensors are what detects various small amounts of chemical vapors.

5.4.4 Wireless Data Collection

Sensor networks are self-configured, wireless, infrastructure-less networks used to measure several conditions such as temperature, pressure, and motion. The collective data are all sent to networks' main infrastructure, where it can be analyzed. The place where the analysis is carried out is called base station. In the wireless network, data is gathered from the base station [31]. The base station is connected through the Internet to share and update the data for later purposes.

Server nodes are present in a WSN as an onboard processor that helps to manage and observe the environment in certain conditions. It acts as a processing unit in the wireless sensor networks system. WSNs can also help to process and analyze the data. Efficient features are data storage and data mining. A collection of sensing devices is connected to communicate with each other. To achieve the interconnection between the network, the server nodes play a vital role in this architecture (Figure 5.7). Sensor network is a structure that has large number of sensor nodes. This network can eliminate the overlapping and implosion, it has a smaller structure, it enables to access the physical environment, and is also energy efficient [32].

Transport Layer	Uploading pre-processed and secured data to the cloud
Security Layer	Encryption/Decryption, privacy and integrity measures
Temporary storage Layer	Data distribution, replication and de-duplication
Pre-Processing Layer	Data analysis, data filtering, reconstruction, and trimming
Monitoring Layer	Activities monitoring, power monitoring, resource monitoring, response monitoring
Physical and virtualization Layer	Virtal sensors and virtual sensors network Things and physical sensors wireless sensor network

Figure 5.7 Wireless sensor network architecture.

5.4.5 Wireless Routing Techniques

There are certain standards for maintaining the protocol for the routing strategy. Networks may differ in their characteristics. The Wireless Routing Protocol has nodes that send the data to their neighbor node; in case of node failure, the neighbor node will be used to retrieve the lost data [13]. TBRPF (Topology Dissemination Based on Reverse-Path Forwarding) is a protocol where every node in the network has the entire information of the topology, and there are many ways to achieve the destination from several paths.

Wireless sensor networks contain hundreds or thousands of these sensor nodes. These sensors have the ability to communicate either among each other or directly to an external base station; because of these advantages WSN is preferred over radio waves, infrared, and optical media. In order to achieve maximum performance and consume less energy, the sensors should be utilized in a proper way.

5.5 Vital Signs Monitoring

5.5.1 Pulse Oxygenation

The term "oxygenation" means addition of oxygen to any chemical or physical system; the instrument used to measure oxygenation is known as pulse oximeter. It is the device that measures the oxygen saturation level or oxygen level present in our blood. The changes are all noted in a graph-like

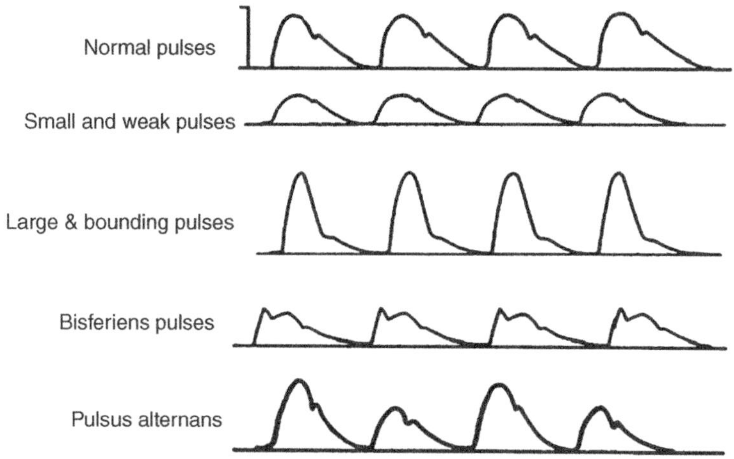

Figure 5.8 Readings of pulse oximetry.

manner; the higher peaks denote a high level of oxygenation (Figure 5.8). An oximeter is a small device with a chip that can be attached to our body [3]. Normally, the reading is all taken from different body parts such as toes, earlobes, and the fingers. The main reason to check these levels is to check whether the heart is pumping the blood properly to all our body parts. Patients who are affected by diseases such as asthma, lung cancer, or heart disease have a high chance of low blood oxygenation levels. Pulse oxygenation is normally measured by SpO2, peripheral capillary oxygen saturation. For a healthy person the level of SpO2 is above 95%, and when the saturation level of SpO2 is less than 90%, it indicates low saturation, which needs an emergency clinical intervention.

An oximeter is an instrument that consists of two main parts, namely, light emitting diodes (LEDs) and a light detector (photodetector). A light beam is passed through the tissue from one side of the probe to the other side. Emitted light is absorbed by the blood and tissues of the part where the oximeter is placed. The amount of light absorbed by the blood varies according to the oxygen saturation of the hemoglobin. On the other hand, the light detector detects the light transmitted from the blood and through the tissue and calculates the values of oxygen saturation (SpO2) [33]. Figure 5.8 defines the different pulse oxygenation levels. A gram of hemoglobin combines with 1.34 ml of oxygen. Normal hemoglobin concentration level is 15 g/dl. The probe is the most delicate part, and damage can be easily made; for purposes of compatibility the rubber probes are preferred and they are robust. The probe connector has a series of a few pins that are connected to the microcontroller. Pulse detection alarms are also a kind of trigger to warn the emergency services.

5.5.2 Blood Pressure

High blood pressure is a common health condition that affects one third of the population. It arises when the pressure exerted by the circulating blood on blood vessels is excessive. It is measured as the systolic number first, followed by the diastolic number. The pressure in the arteries at the time of contraction of the heart muscle is called systolic pressure, and the minimum pressure during relaxation and dilation of the ventricles of the heart is called diastolic pressure. These two pressure numbers are very prominent to determine the health of the heart. The greater the number than its ideal range, the harder the heart is trying to pump blood to other parts of our body. For a normal, healthy heart, the systolic pressure is in the range 90 to 120 and the diastolic pressure in the range 60 to 80. Readings are expressed in millimeters of mercury, abbreviated mmHg. Normal readings of blood pressure are below 120/80 mmHg and above the 90/60 mmHg in a healthy adult condition. Readings greater than 120/80 mmHg are considered a red flag. The higher blood pressure levels lead to a higher risk of having other health problems, such as heart disease, heart attack, and stroke [34–35].

The measurements are read form the instrument, and then the pressure is calculated based on an algorithm. Blood pressure monitoring systems use wireless technology making home monitoring of patients easier and improves the relationship between doctor and patient. These devices offer regular online monitoring for a patient that proposes more enhanced diagnosis as well as improved efficiency and quality of administration even during the absence of doctor. Other than this, ultrasonic techniques are also incorporated in blood pressure devices; in this technique, blood pressure is measured from the blood vessel by performing transmission of an ultra sonic wave and reception of a reflected wave with respect to the blood vessel using an ultrasonic probe.

This technique can be implemented in an anklet to obtain the end result (Figure 5.9). In remote areas this is mainly used to track the patient's medical condition; for this, an accurate and reliable measurement sensor has to be perfectly selected. One device can measure various parameters such as arterial pressure and pulse rate. It needs to be mostly accurate and the data transmitted to the cloud server, for monitoring purposes.

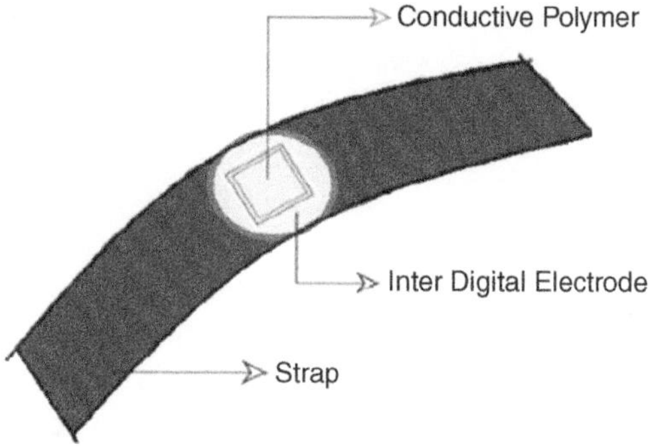

Figure 5.9 Working of blood pressure sensor.

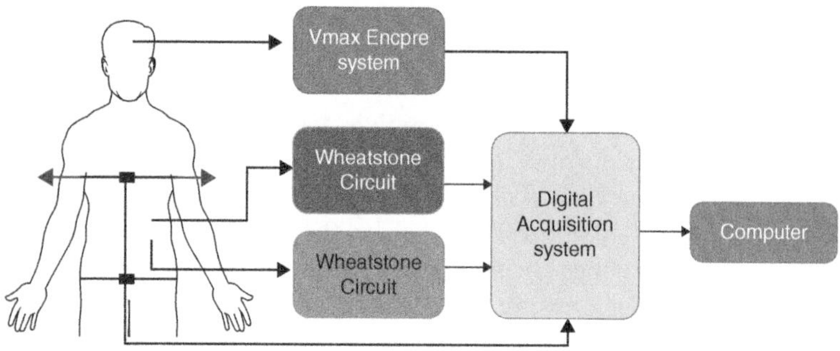

Figure 5.10 Measurement of respiration rate.

5.5.3 Respiration Rate

Respiration rate is a physiological measurement in a patient's observation. As in several cases of acidosis, this will be important information for healthcare. In severe illnesses, the respiration rate is one of the most sensible indications such as in case of potential hypoxia and distress. There are several methods to measure the respiration rate such as the piezoelectric sensor method, laser Doppler, vibrometer method, pyroelectric transducer method, impedance pneumography method, capnography method, and photoplethysmography (PPG) signal [36]. The chest volume variation during inhaling and exhaling is normally collected to form the respiratory wave. This technology is based on a loop wire with constant current that generates a magnetic field proportional to the loop orientation of the vest (Figure 5.10). In relaxed normal breathing the respiratory rate is 12–20 breaths per minute. Chest expansion on inspiration should be the same or similar on each breath. The measurement procedure has been already demonstrated to precisely monitor cardiac activity.

This system comprises (i) a magnet and (ii) a sensor, which includes a coil made of magnetic microwire whose sensor coil is configured to detect motion of the magnet relative to the magnetic sensor coil, wherein the magnetic microwire sensor coil is oriented such that field lines emanating from the magnet are parallel to a cross-sectional area of the magnetic microwire sensor coil and the magnetic microwire sensor coil winding direction. The sensor is positioned at a distance from the magnet such that the magnetic microwire sensor coil is magnetically coupled to the magnet.

5.5.4 Heart Rate

Heart rate (HR) is one of the main information variables in health and fitness activity. Information of heart rate cycle provides the physiological changes by monitoring its signal regularly. Its signals can be easily obtained from the ECG and PPG signals. These two signals have their information in waveform and contain similar heart rate information. It is crucial to analyze how the heart reacts during exercise and other sports activities (Table 5.2). The activities help to evaluate the heart rate variability. This analysis is a simple indicator of the cardiovascular system [15]. Pulse signals measurements are related to heart rate that can be used in this method. It is defined as the palpable rhythmic expansion of an artery produced by the increase in volume of blood pushed into the vessel caused by contraction and relaxation of the heart. This information gives more than the heart rate and includes variables such as amplitude, strength, and regularity of pulse. There are two types of PPG:

- **Transmission:** Light transmitted from the device will enter through any vascular part of the body such as an earlobe and the detector will receive the signal.
- **Reflection:** Light emitted from the device will get reflected from some parts of the body.

Table 5.2 Heart rate comparison table.

Heart rate	Effort	Effect
171–190	90–100%	Develops maximum performance and speed.
152–171	80–90%	Increase maximum performance capacity.
133–152	70–80%	Improves aerobic fitness
144–133	60–70%	Improves basic endurance and fat burning
95–114	50–60%	Improves overall health and helps recovery

The heartbeat sensor contains a light-emitting diode and a detector such as a photodiode. Blood flow in our body is caused by the heartbeat pulses. When the tissue in our body is illuminated with some light source, such as an LED, it either reflects or transmits the light [41]. Some of the emitted light is absorbed by the blood circulating in the tissue and some is transmitted. The reflected light from the blood is received by the light detector. Blood volume in the tissue is indicated by the amount of light absorbed. The detected output is proportional to the heartbeat rate and is in the form of an electrical signal. This signal is a DC signal related to the blood volume and tissues, and the AC component is synchronous with the heartbeat and causes some changes in blood volume [42]. The main requirement is to isolate the AC component.

5.5.5 Body Temperature

Body temperature is the measurement of the balance with heat produced and loss of heat in the body. Body temperature is measured to avoid many dysfunctionalities due to excessive temperature. Body temperature is measured by two methods, core temperature (CT) and skin temperature (ST). While the body's thermoregulation mechanism regulates core body temperature, skin temperature varies in a wider range [37]. Skin temperature is affected by blood circulation and is also related with heart rate and metabolic rate. Other factors such as air circulation, humidity, and ambient temperature also play a major role in the body temperature regulation system.

Temperature sensing can be done by directly heating the source or with the source being heated through radiated energy, remotely. There are a large variety of temperature sensing devices, such as thermocouples, thermistors, infrared, resistance temperature detectors (RTDs), and semiconductor sensors.

Radiation temperature detector sensors are one of the most accurate sensing devices. In a radiation temperature detector, resistance is directionally proportional to the temperature (Figure 5.11). A radiation temperature detector is made of nickel, platinum, and copper. Temperature measuring capability can be used to measure accurate temperature in the range between −270 and +850 °C. There are unique techniques to measure the temperature by using the radiation temperature detector [38]:

- In the two-wired method, a current is forced and the resulting voltage is measured. The main advantage of this method is that is simple to connect and implement, and its drawback is it has noise interference; because of that it leads to measurement errors.

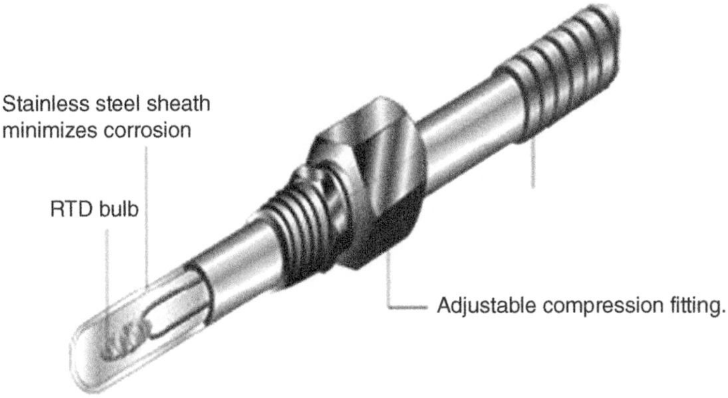

Figure 5.11 Measuring body temperature.

- The three-wired method is similar to the two-wired method, but the third wire compensates for the lead resistance.
- In the four-wired method, the current is forced on the wires and the voltage is sensed on the other set of wires.

5.5.6 Blood Glucose

Blood glucose is the main sugar found in your blood. It comes from the food you eat and is your body's main source of energy. For a living body, the main source of energy is blood glucose for cell activity. It is important to maintain a stable concentration of glucose present in the blood, and homeostatic systems tightly regulate the glucose level.

Many diabetic people do not feel significant symptoms, unless they experience hyperglycemia, which makes glucose level too high, or hypoglycemia, which makes glucose level too low [39]. Hyperglycemia might cause crucial damage to some organs, which may lead to complications. This includes some other symptoms:

- Heart attack or stroke (cardiac or vascular event);
- Kidney problems, which may require dialysis;
- Eye problems, which cause loss of vision;
- Sexual issues such as erectile dysfunction;
- Problems with circulation and scarring (amputation).

A CGM (continuous glucose monitor) is used to measure the glucose found in the fluid between the cells in your body (Figure 5.12). Using tiny

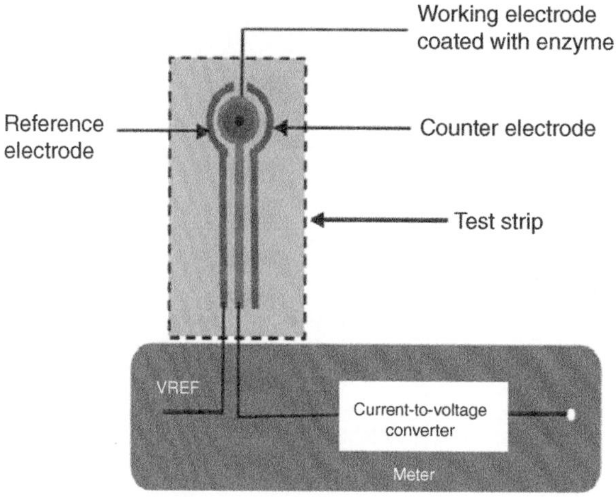

Figure 5.12 Schematic diagram of CGM.

sensors, many devices collect information in their own manner. Sometimes, the sensor is placed at the top of our stomach for a quick result without any pain or can be adhered to the back of our arm. The information is sent by the transmitter, which is present on the sensor, to a wireless monitor system that you can clip on your belt. The sugar level is displayed at 5-, 10-, or 15-minutes intervals [40]. If our sugar level drops to a dangerous low or high preset level, the system will sound the alarm. Continuous glucose monitoring will give a clear image of the glucose highs and lows. This means we will be able to see trends and the impact of any given meal as well as gaining insight on our glucose levels.

5.6 Biosensors in M-Health

The use of smart technologies in medicine and healthcare has been steadily increasing over the last years. Health and well-being monitoring systems are now deployed in homes, at work, and in everyday environments to support health, smart homes, and age-friendly workplaces. Smart sensors and medical devices of a large variety are used to support physical and behavioral monitoring, as well as to show interaction with social aspects of daily routine. They focus on particular health conditions or on the more social aspects of well-being and good quality of life. However, still there are several technology and societal challenges that prevent smart biosensors from widespread adoption and deployment.

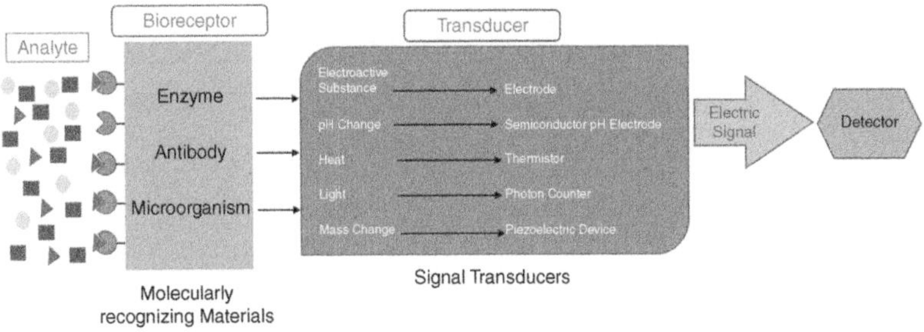

Figure 5.13 Bio sensors- bio signals to electric signals.

These are mainly related to cost, integrity, and scalability. However, there is a need to process the large amount of data collected from sensors. These sensors may operate either as direct or as indirect sensors, often referred to homogeneous and heterogeneous immunosensors, respectively [49] (Figure 5.13). Biosensors are firmly established for application in clinical chemical analysis.

Biosensors have been used widely throughout the world for glucose testing at home, bringing diagnosis to on-site analysis. Information is further analyzed to obtain the evidence needed to offer personalized interventions that support smart living and provide better health.

The second solution presents an IoT ecosystem that combines sensors embedded in smart health wearables with mobile and static devices to improve occupational safety and health, provide personalized recommendations that benefit physical and mental health, and improve workforce productivity.

Finally, the third solution focuses on the development of an intelligent non-invasive biosignal-recording system to detect the condition and analyze infants during sleep.

5.6.1 Bioresorbable Biosensors

Implantable biosensors are an important class of biosensors because of their ability to provide continuous data on the levels of a target analyte. They enable changes in analyte levels over time to be monitored without any need for intervention from either the patient or clinician. These implantable medical devices have great potential in the diagnosis, monitoring, management, and treatment of a variety of disease conditions. This trend addresses medium-term needs of medical applications and germinates from former efforts on compatibility and degradability of materials used in compatible implantation of devices for chronical diseases [50]. Materials that dissolve fully in the body with biological by-products provide the only method to create separate optical, electrical, and sensing components to implantable biodegradable systems that eliminate any boundary with the human body.

5.6.2 Electrochemical Biosensors

An electrochemical bio sensor may even be an integrated device that is capable of providing specific quantitative association degree and analytical information using a biological recognition part. A number of different types of electrochemical biosensors exist depending on their method for ensuring biological selectivity or their signal transduction method. The receptor can be selective for a biocatalytic event such as a reaction that is catalyzed by macromolecules, including enzymes, or for a specific bioaffinity, such as the interaction between an analyte and a macromolecule, independent of their biological environment [51]. Electrochemical biosensors are also robust, easy to miniaturize, and offer broad detection limits even when only small volumes of analyte are present.

5.6.3 Enzymatic Biosensors

The enzyme biosensor is composed of a sensitive membrane-immobilized enzyme and electrode transducer system, which combine an enzyme and the electrode together. It has advantages of both high stability of insoluble enzyme system and the high sensitivity of electrochemical systems [52]. Biosensors allow the analysis in complicated biological media. The detection of a large range of compounds is used in various kinds of research and in food management industries. It's conjointly indispensable within the healthcare field for the diagnosis and later treatment of diseases and watching of diseases. The biotechnology and pharmaceutical industries greatly want frequent to continuous analysis of biological media.

5.6.4 FET Biosensors

The field-effect transistor-based biosensor, also called biosensor field-effect transistor (Bio-FET), may even be a field-effect transistor that is formed by binding of the molecules, and it changes within the surface. Once the molecules get charged, the biomolecules bind to the field-effect transistor gate. They are going to stop the charge distribution of the underlying semiconductor leading to amendment in the electric field effect transistor channel. The Bio-FET consists of two important compartments: first is that the biological recognizing part. The Bio-FET is essentially supported by the ion-sensitive transistor (ISFET), a kind of metal oxide semiconductor transistor (MOSFET) where the inner metallic gate is replaced by an associate degree ion-sensitive membrane [53]. Due to binding of the analyte, the operation of Bio-FET devices support for detection of fields such as food analysis and medical diagnostics. This identical mechanism of glass conductor sensor that conjointly sight changes in surface potential. Because of the little magnitude of the changes in surface potential upon binding of biomolecule or dynamical hydrogen ion concentration, glass electrodes need a high electric resistance electronic equipment that will increase the dimensions and value of the device.

5.6.5 Flexible and Wearable Biosensors

Flexible and versatile wearable biosensors have more potential to attach to the skin and extract bio-fluids for real-time and continuous watching of physical activities. Wearable sensors strengthen the resource property by collecting data periodically and it can also be used remotely. These adaptable, easy, battery-free, non-invasive devices incessantly and it will monitor the user's well-being and transfer information wirelessly. They need a good potential to boost quality of life with timely in medical domain and therefore early treatments [54]. To improve the accuracy of signal monitoring and diagnosis and user comfort, certain exploration and improvements are made on materials, power consumption, life of wearable devices. We tend to classify wearable biosensors by sensing medical conditions like heart rate, sweat aldohexose, neural structure shunt flow and ototoxic chemicals and discuss challenges and prospects for those flexible and wearable biosensors.

5.6.6 Metal Oxide Biosensors

Metal Oxide–based electrodes offer a biocompatible electroactive surface for catalyst immobilization with improved conformation, orientation, and biological activity. Detection systems for monitoring air and water quality using metal oxides are of great interest to improve the selectivity and sensitivity of current sensing devices, and at the same time allowing simultaneous measurements of numerous parameters with real-time response. These devices to be commercially viable, they must be stable during operation, with a uniform and reproducible signal for a prolonged period of time, despite being able to precisely detect a specific gas even in mixtures of different gases. As a result, it cannot change the enzymes or reduce at the conductor surface.

The chance of direct lepton transmission between enzymes based on NMO conductor surface can pave the approach for the event of superior reagent less bio sensing devices, which should obviate those requirements for mediators, permitting economical transduction of bio recognition events. Al-doped ZnO (AZO) electrodes have better stability at the progression and also add the fabrication of photoconductors using ultraviolet and nanowires with ZnO [55]. On the other hand, the deposition of CuO on AZO electrodes shows rectifying behavior related to the p-type conduction in CuO. The structure is with diode-to-diode formation including the n-type electrodes. In contrast to ZnO photoconductors, these structures present illumination with visible optical response and infrared light as well as short turn-on and recovery time.

5.6.7 Micro Fluidic Biosensors

Microfluidics could also be generalized by the term and separate or along fluid behavior, specific management, and manipulation at the sub-millimeter scale. Micro-fluidic systems offer outturn process, enhanced transport for dominant flow conditions, increased mixing rate of varied agents [56]. It offers fundamentally new capabilities in the control of concentrations of molecules in space and time. The material most commonly adopted for the fabrication of microfluidic structures is poly-dimethylsiloxane. The integration of microfluidic device and biosensor technologies provides new opportunities for biosensing applications, such as portability, real-time detection, increased sensitivity and selectivity. By integrating the microfluidic structures, sample processing and biosensing reactions are carried out within a closed and relatively stable environment, thus promising better sensitivity and reliability. These devices are capable of automation It enables delivering of various kinds of samples in sequential orders can be realized by unique design of microfluid channels, pneumatic valves.

5.6.8 Polymer Organic Biosensors

Conducting Polymers are used to enhance speed, sensitivity and versatility of biosensors in diagnostics to measure vital analytes. Various carriers that are considered as immobilizing enzymes, conducting polymer, hydrogel materials, chitin, and chitosan offer most of the characteristics that are mentioned above. Enzymatic redox reaction composition of the binder and the immobilization matrix is based on the biomaterials and biocatalysts, solid supports electron transport mediators, as electron collectors within constructions of the enzyme electrode is critical to get optimum current from the enzymatic redox reactions. The proper use of different polymer materials is entirely influenced by the redox reactions and electron transportation kinetics of the enzyme electrodes. Conducting polymers are known to be compatible with biological molecules in neutral aqueous solutions and it have the ability to efficiently transfer electric charge produced by the biochemical reaction to electronic circuit.

5.7 IoT-Based Rehabilitation System

The IoT is the next technological innovation; the advancements in artificial intelligence and machine learning have made the automation of IoT devices easy. The main problems are the aging demographics and a scarcity of healthcare staff; sensible systems on IoT are getting a safer way to solve these problems. The use of IoT technology alone can establish an information network that interconnects hospitals, communities, healthcare devices increase the response time for the patient. This technology permits computers to improve and perceive the symptoms and medical services, permitting them to create a recovery arrange and fast reconfigure medical resources consistent with the distinctive wants of the patient. In the meantime, IoT offers a lot interconnection of all resources and providing instant engagement in data through the cloud. IoT consists of a collection of technologies that enable a large variety of appliances, devices, and objects to act with one another and communicate with the other networking technologies. Devices are usually the active item in IoT that provide the small connections. There are several IoT applications, as well as healthcare, industrial, and bus systems. Attention systems use a collection of interconnected devices to form an IoT network dedicated to attention analysis, as well as patient observation and automatic detection of things wherever medical interventions are needed. The general system collects data from numerous sensing devices through a middleware that provides the ability and protection needed for attention within the context of IoT (Figure 5.14). Using IoT technology alone will produce a data network that connects hospitals, communities, attention devices, homes, and different terminals. The network have access to the monitoring devices that detect the bio-signals of the patients in real-time, a home gateway that is responsible for data analysis and forward sensing data to the remote server [45]. There are still two key issues in applying IoT-based rehabilitation: (i) patient speedy diagnosis; and (ii) diagnostic-based reconfiguration of rehabilitation strategy and rehabilitation resources. Ontology, which remains to be explored, is found to be a promising approach

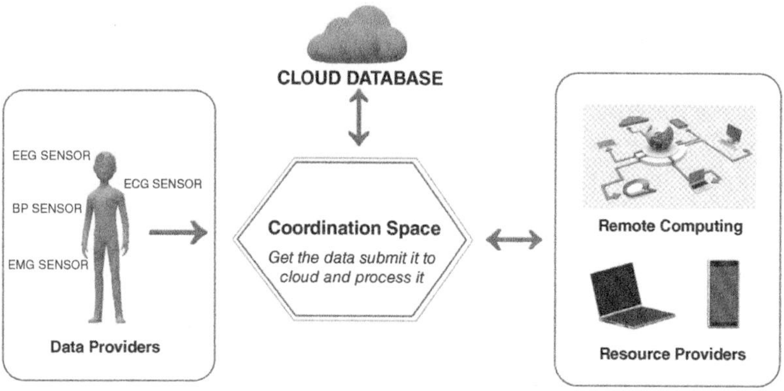

Figure 5.14 Block diagram of IOT rehabilitation system.

to facilitate noticing an answer for such a large-scale system quickly as IoT-based rehabilitation system [44]. However, its goal is to fulfill the necessities of a designer mistreatment process strategies.

The usage of in IoT frameworks in rehabilitation engineering shows two main advantages over traditional approaches. First, metaphysics provides higher organized domain data concerning recovery engineering, which permits hospitals to try and do higher analysis with a straightforward relationship of inclusion, parallel relationship, and fewer or no clarifications. The combination of IoT technology and metaphysics would enable acceptable care and therefore the best configuration of the medical resources to be found. Second, applying metaphysics permits a higher exchange of data. A system is developed that mixes IoT with metaphysics to produce speedy and economic recovery for various patients. Experimental results on lower limb rehabilitation show that the planned IoT-based rehabilitation system will perform properly, and therefore the ontology-based method (the application of which is still at exploring stage, is found as a promising attempt that can help to quickly find the solution for such large-scale system), which facilitates developing a good rehabilitation strategy and reconfigure all resources quickly consistent with the need. Wi-Fi and RFID-based short-distance radio communication technologies GPS-based location technology, (UID-(Unique Identifier)based) technology, and service-oriented design (SOA)-based design technology can be used to establish a rehabilitation system.

The SOA is employed as a basis for planning, implementing, deploying, invoking, and managing attention services. The system topology includes all medical resources (e.g., hospitals, rehabilitation center, doctors, nurses, ambulances, and medical devices), communities and patients, and a server with information, as well as an accountable intermediate process for information analysis, consolidation, rehabilitation strategy creation, and demanding events detection. Throughout the outlined network, these devices are interconnected by a LAN with the Transmission Control Protocol and the Internet Protocol (TCP/IP) and every one of the devices is assigned a UID. Throughout the meantime, RFID tags monitor and approve the physicians, nurses, patients, and different human resources.

ADM (Automating Design Methodology) with ontology-based resource reconfiguration is applied to make subsystems of rehabilitation quickly and expeditiously consistent with a patient's specific demands. A typical rehabilitation subsystem planned is sometimes composed of a sensible rehabilitation system that gives the most rehabilitation treatment, sensible observance devices that notice patients' bio-signals in real time, a home entrance for information analysis and transmission of sensed information to the remote server, and an sensing camera that monitors the patient and doctors or nurses. Wi-Fi links the system devices to an entrance device to make a LAN, and therefore the subsystem may communicate with others or the wide space network (WAN) via the regular entrance device protocol. Thus GPS, which is incorporated into the medical system, gathers location data. That way, enclosed by a lot of educated population that uses communication and data technology, patients and medical workers will notice redoubled opportunities for acceptable home care.

5.7.1 Automating Methodology in IOT Framework

There are three stages within the interaction interface design process. These stages are responsible for communicating with the data servers and the human interactions (Figure 5.15). All these levels are further composed of various sub-blocks, and each unit processes the output of another stage to provide an optimized output. The connection is established through the IoT by wireless communication techniques, such as Wi-Fi and Bluetooth [46].

5.7.2 Diagnosis Processing

The diagnostic process is a complex transition process that begins with the patient's individual illness history and culminates in a result that can be categorized by using automated methodologies it becomes easier. Patient health conditions are checked by the doctors and treated for the required symptoms of the disease. Such variables are categorized into three categories and eight subclasses. The three categories are basic patient data with subclasses based on the patient's age and gender, and alternative connected

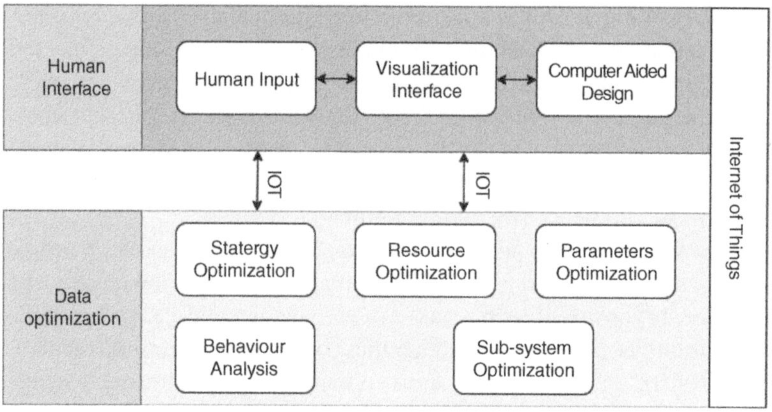

Figure 5.15 Framework of rehabilitation system methodology.

data with subclasses such as length of unwellness. All this data is gathered are stored in the database system to provide remote access to that information for any future purpose.

In the meantime, predicted actions, which means the specified result that we would like from the tool for recovery, are often obtained from the need. After that, we have a tendency to understand the tailored preferences just like the lowest price or best care. The connections between the individual and the disease are all tracked to avoid the condition in future cases. Optimization of the data is an essential role in transmitting different kinds of information.

5.7.3 Rehabilitation Strategy Design

Therapeutic plan design is required after the first stage in order to figure out the best therapeutic approach for patients. Two essential tasks have to be completed during this process. Next, with the aid of strategic optimization, more comprehensive therapy plans need to be carried out. In this phase the circumstances of the patients are paired with the database reports to tackle the disease to track the common cases for the particular symptoms. There are some effective strategies and comprehensive recovery plans that will be used in such conditional terms, such as the needed treatment for the patient such as to maintain the health condition as stabilized by taking regular walking as a practice and the session details all included in the informational database system.

Tasks are evaluated from the design purposes; it's possible to include the specified functions and fulfill the initial specifications. The second phase, designing the strategy of the design phase systems, offers medical services for the selected patients in the rehabilitation system from the previous section. The recovery measures are calculated from the rehabilitation strategy. Additionally to the relevant procedure, the metaphysics of the medical resource also includes data concerning every medical resource. The assignment of the resources is carried out depending on the collected data. Data are provided with a certain interval of time so the flow of design will remain consistent.

The distribution methods are the most effective or the best ones that are consistent with the patient's urgent needs. Nonetheless, there is a certain expected difference in the real-time systems and the original modules action by the arrangement. Certain strategies are employed to improve the result accuracy for betterment of patient health conditions.

5.7.4 Subsystem Design

When a patient got recovered by using the strategy design that has rehabilitation plans, it provides a details overview of the medical issue of patient and his/her medical recovery strategy in a workflow. However, a patient is taken care of by associate degree IoT-based recovery program. Conflicts will occur once various patients needed to put together use a similar machine to train on their basics, at a similar location in step with the therapeutic technique being recommended. A similar conclusion is true of all the tools for recovery and alternative associated programs.

As a result, in the improving process, certain optimization is needed because the entire system construction reaches the third level. Theoretically, the delivered optimization is similar to the obtained resources, planned changes are reflected in the results. Altering the device alone helps to fix the major problems' it's vital to revive either the configuration or perhaps the feature model. Through this manner, repetition ensures the resulted curative effect.

5.7.5 Detail Design

In the design process in which the arrangement, forms, dimensions, and duration of all of the individual activities are finally arranged, the equipment is specified, treatment schedules are assessed, costs are estimated. Optimization of parameters is important to ensure that the specifications meet the structure requirements [47–48]. This is the level to which knowledge integration and application integration are implemented in the recovery framework with technical support from the component components

Class Mapping Data Transformation Technique and Component Object Model/Distribution Component Object Model (COM/DCOM).

Such integration is desperately needed since the program mentioned above is focused not only on the databases with detailed content on the basic patient and disease information and device role definition and service status but also on the knowledge base on disease diagnosis and treatment strategy [43] (Figure 5.16). Both of these must be deeply integrated in the recovery process [46] so that the program can function properly. This is also important to design coordination. Project management and operational management laid the groundwork for integration to ensure that the project is conducted in the right direction.

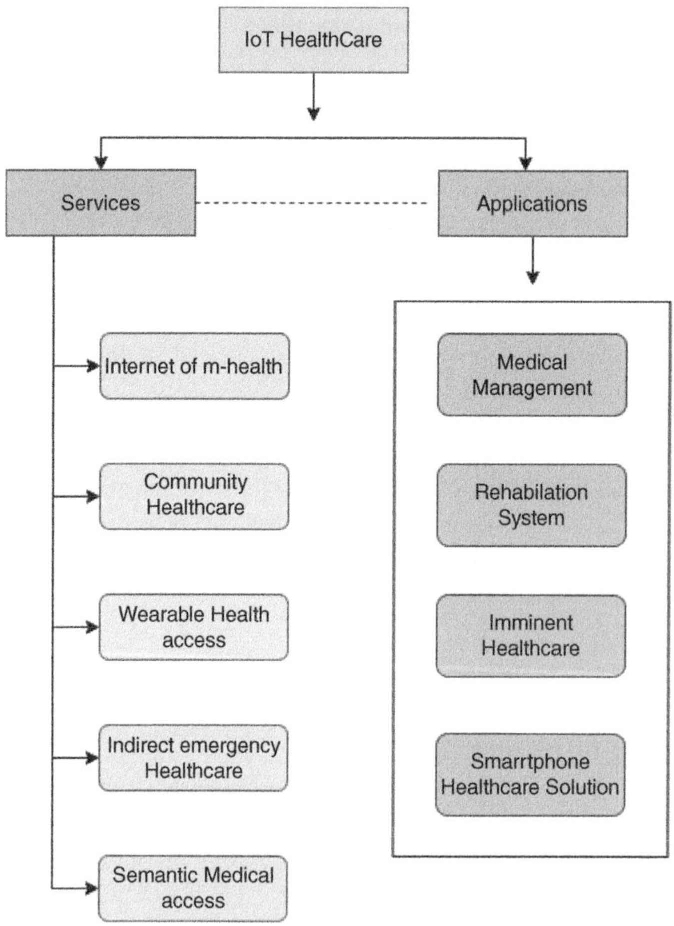

Figure 5.16 Services and applications of IOT.

5.7.6 Security in IoT

IoT protection has become a problem for enterprises because without a robust security architecture, large volumes of data flowing and being stored through the networks are exposed to infrastructure vulnerabilities that hackers can exploit. For those cyber threats and hacking, the security, integrity, and availability of data must be protected through the IT infrastructure. Mechanisms or methods for safe data exchange, storage, and sharing including the use of the new cryptographic methods or encryption algorithms should be introduced.

5.8 Future Work

In healthcare, IoT offers multiple benefits. According to several reports, the implementation of IoT in the healthcare system will considerably improve by the end of 2022; experts have predicted that it will reach 74 billion wearable technology around the globe by 2025. With the recent feature of cloud computing, data from sensors are directly updated in the IoT and so they are highly accessible.

5.9 Conclusion

Implementing the proposed system, waiting times in the hospitals will all be reduced, resulting in less time wasted for many people. This works remotely, so the patients' live location is also accessible via the sensor modules. Doctors can have complete control of their patients' medical records, and monitoring has improved to track their health status. Prevention is better than cure, and diseases are early diagnosed, which leads to preventing deadlier diseases. Error occurrence is minimal by using digitalized sensors. It saves huge costs of medical expenses. The security of data is also a vital factor, which will improve in upcoming decades.

Authors' Biography

M. Saravanan received his B.E. degree in electrical and electronics from Coimbatore Institute of Technology-Coimbatore, India, in 2006 and his masters in VLSI design from Anna University Coimbatore in 2009. After

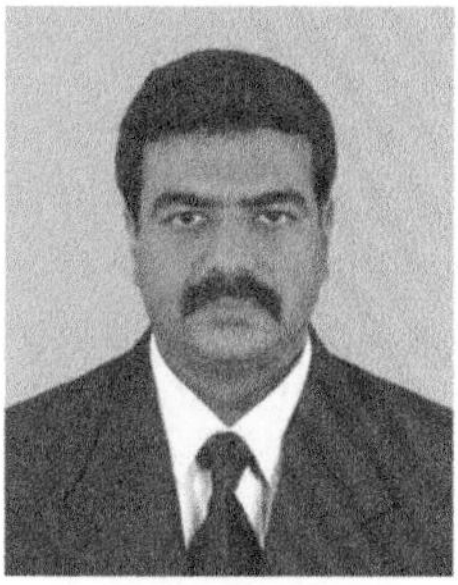

graduation, he has 11 years of teaching experience, and now he is working as an assistant professor in the Department of Electronics and Communication Engineering at Sri Eshwar College of Engineering, Coimbatore, India. His research includes VLSI design, nano-electronics, and semiconductor devices. He is also a member of IEEE EDS and IEEE Photonics society. Email: saranecedgl@gmail.com.

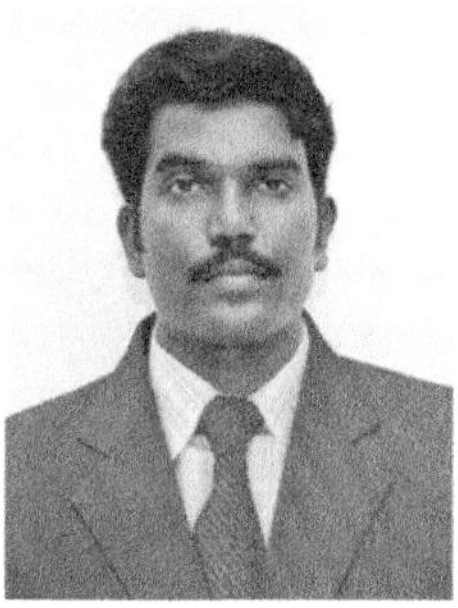

J. Ajayan received the B.Tech. degree in electronics and communication engineering from Kerala University, Trivandrum, India, in 2009, the M. Tech. degree in VLSI design from Karunya University, Coimbatore, India, in 2012, and the PhD degree in electronics and communication engineering from Karunya University, Coimbatore, India, in 2017. He is an associate professor in the Department of Electronics and Communication Engineering at SR University, Warangal, Telangana, India. He is author of many refereed international journals (Elsevier, Taylor and Francis, Springer, IOP Science).

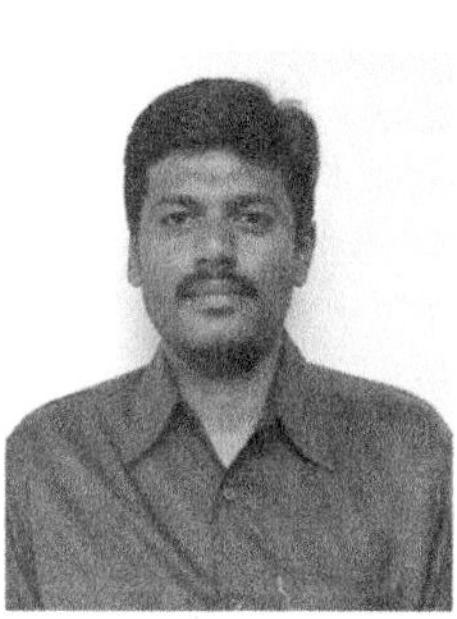

R. Maheswar has completed his B.E. (ECE) from Madras University in 1999, M.E. (Applied Electronics) from Bharathiyar University in 2002, and PhD in the field of wireless sensor networks from Anna University in 2012. He has about 19 years of teaching experience at various levels and is presently working as an associate professor in the School of EEE, VIT Bhopal University, Bhopal, Madhya Pradesh, India. He has published 70 papers at international journals and international conferences. His research interests include wireless sensor networks, queueing theory, and performance evaluation.

Dr. Eswaran Parthasarathy received his bachelor's degree in electronics and telecommunication engineering from the Institute of Engineers (India) in 2000, the masters in mechatronics in 2003 from Madras Institute of Technology (India) and a PhD degree in electronics and communication engineering from SRM University in 2014. He is currently an associate professor in SRM Institute of Science and Technology. His areas of interest are MEMS, VLSI, device modeling, EV, PV systems, embedded systems, and industry 4.0. He has published over 30 reviewed international journal/conference papers and two Indian patents. He has served as a reviewer for peer-reviewed journals. He is also fellow member of IE (India), life member of IETE and ISTE professional bodies. Email: eswaranp@srmist.edu.in.

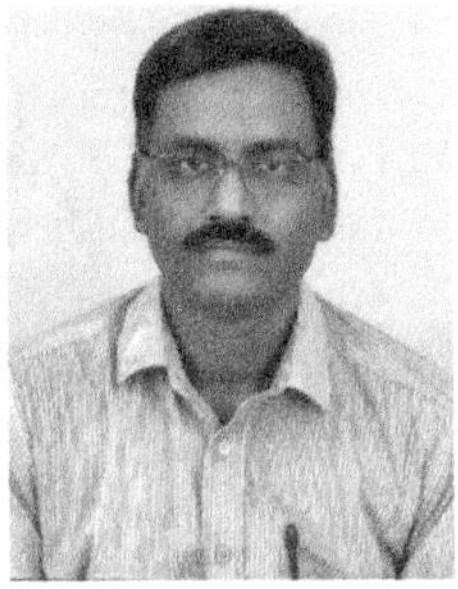

References

1 Abdullah, A., Ismael, A., Rashid, A., Abou-ElNour, A. and Tarique, M. (2015). "Real Time Wireless Health Monitoring Application using Mobile Devices", 3.

2 Aminian, M. and Naji, H.R. (2013). "A Hospital Healthcare Monitoring System Using Wireless Sensor Networks,", Department of Computer, Science and Research branch, Islamic Azad University, Kerman, Iran and College of Electrical and Computer Engineering, Kerman Graduate University of Technology, Iran, Vol 4.

3 Bhoomika, B.K. and Muralidhara, K.N. (2015). Secured smart healthcare monitoring system based on IoT. *International Journal on Recent and Innovation Trends in Computing and Communication* 3 (7): 4958–4961.

4 Anbumani, S., Kavin, R., Saranya, A. et al. (2015). An intelligent patient tele-monitoring system using android technology. *International Journal of Research in Engineering and Technology* 4 (2): 477–482.

5 Kassanos, P., Ip, H.M.D., and Yang, G. (2015). A tetrapolar bio-impedance sensing system for gastrointestinal tract monitoring. In: *2015 IEEE 12th International Conference on Wearable and Implantable Body Sensor Networks (BSN)*, 1–6. https://doi.org/10.1109/BSN.2015.7299403.

6 Swamy, G., Kodali, R.K., and Lakshmi, B. (2015). "An Implementation of IoT for Healthcare", IEEE Recent Advances in Intelligent Computational Systems (RAICS) 10–12 December 2015.

7 Catarinucci, L. et al. (2015). An IoT-aware architecture for smart healthcare systems. *IEEE Internet of Things Journal* 2 (6): 515–526. https://doi.org/10.1109/JIOT.2015.2417684.

8 Gupta, P., Agrawal, D., Chhabra, J., Dhir, P.K. (2016). "IoT based Smart HealthCare Kit", Jaypee University of Information Technology, International Conference on Computational Techniques in Information and Communication Technologies (ICCTICT).

9 Sivakanth, T. and Sathish, K. (2016). Design of Iot based smart health monitoring and alert system. 9: 7655–7661.

10 Tai, B., Hung, K., and Zhan, Y.T. (2004). Wearable medical devices for tele-home healthcare. *IEMBS'04. 26th Annual International Conference of the IEEE* 2: 5384–5387.

11 Shamim Hossain, M. and Muhammad, G. (2016). Cloud-assisted industrial internet of things (IIoT)–enabled framework for health monitoring. *Computer Networks* 101: 192–202.

12 Xia, H., Asif, I., and Zhao, X. (2013). Cloud-ECG for real time ECG monitoring and analysis. *Computer Methods and Programs in Biomedicine* 110 (3): 253–259.

13 Jassas, M.S., Qasem, A.A., and Mahmoud, Q.H. (2015). A smart system connecting e-health sensors and the cloud. In: *Electrical and Computer Engineering (CCECE), 2015 IEEE 28th Canadian Conference*, 712–716. IEEE.

14 Thilakanathan, D., Chen, S., Nepal, S. et al. (2014). A platform for secure monitoring and sharing of generic health data in the Cloud. *Future Generation Computer Systems* 35: 102–113.

15 Adivarekar, J.S., Chordia, A.D., Baviskar, H.H., Aher, P.V. and Gupta, S. (2013), "Patient Monitoring System Using GSM Technology", 2 March 2013.

16 Murray, A. and Khambete, N.D. (2012). National efforts to improve healthcare technology management and medical device safety in India. In: *7th International Conference IET*, 1–5.

17 Atalla, S., Aziz, K., Ismail, S.H., and Tarapiah, S. (2016). "Smart real-time healthcare monitoring and tracking system using GSM/GPS technologies", 3rd MEC International Conference on Big Data and Smart City.

18 Lakshmipriya, N., Hariprasath, E., Indrakumar, V. et al. (2017). Automatic patient monitoring system using raspberry Pi-3. *International Journal of Advanced Research in Electrical, Electronics and Instrumentation Engineering* 6 (3).

19 Muralidhara, K.N. and Bhoomika, B.K. Secured smart healthcare monitoring system based on IoT. *International Journal on Recent and Innovation Trends in Computing and Communication* 3 (7).

20 Mahesh Kumar, D. (2012). Healthcare monitoring system using wireless sensor network. *International Journal of Advanced Networking and Applications* 4 (1).

21 Sathe, S. and Kulkarni, A. (2014). Health care applications of the internet of things: a review. *International Journal of Computer Science and Information Technologies (IJCSIT)* 5 (5): 6229–6232.

22 Kumar, R. and Rajasekaran, M.P. (2016). An IoT-based Patient monitoring system using raspberry pi. In: *2016 International Conference on Computing Technologies and Intelligent Data Engineering (ICCTIDE'16)*, 1–4.

23 Tkacz, B., Riitters, K., and Percy, K.E. (2013). Forest monitoring methods in the United States and Canada. *Developments in Environmental Science* 12: 49–73.

24 Al-awlaqi, M.A.A.H., Li, M.S., O'Grady, M. et al. (2018). Wearable IoT enabled real-time health monitoring system. *EURASIP Journal on Wireless Communications and Networking* 2018: 298.

25 Dubey, R.. (2008). System Architecture and Overview Smart Sensors", National Conference on Emerging Trends in Industrial Automation NCEICS-08 at Apeejay college of engineering, Sohna (Gurgaon) on Sept, 27th. 2008.

26 Yunusa, Z., Hamidon, M.N., Kaiser, A., and Awang, Z. (2014). Gas sensors: a review. *Sensors and Transducers* 168: 61–75.

27 Firdaus, N.A., Yulianto, A., and Kusriyanto, M. (2015). Wireless sensor network application for carbon monoxide monitoring. In: *2015 9th International Conference on Telecommunication Systems Services and Applications (TSSA)*, 1–4. Bandung.

28 Sawada, K., Takahashi, K., Iwata, T., and Hattori, T. (2017). CMOS based ion image sensor – fusion of bio sensor technology and image sensor technology. In: *2017 19th International Conference on Solid-State Sensors, Actuators and Microsystems (TRANSDUCERS)*, 131–134. Kaohsiung.

29 Wilson, D. and Shepherd, L. (2008). Chemical and biological sensors for environmental monitoring. In: *2008 IEEE International Symposium on Circuits and Systems*, 1990–1993. Seattle, WA.

30 Plata, M.R., Contento, A.M., and Ríos, A. (2010). State-of-the-art of (bio) chemical sensor developments in analytical Spanish groups. *Sensors (Basel)* 10 (4): 2511–2576.

31 Pinar, Y., Zuhair, A., Hamad, A. et al. (2016). Wireless sensor networks (WSNs). In: *2016 IEEE Long Island Systems, Applications and Technology Conference (LISAT)*, 1–8. Farmingdale, NY.

32 Jino Ramson, S.R. and Moni, D.J. (2017). Applications of wireless sensor networks – a survey. In: *2017 International Conference on Innovations in Electrical, Electronics, Instrumentation and Media Technology (ICEEIMT)*, 325–329. Coimbatore.

33 Perkins, G.D., McAuley, D.F., Giles, S. et al. (2003). Do changes in pulse oximeter oxygen saturation predict equivalent changes in arterial oxygen saturation. *Critical Care Medicine* 7: R67–R71.

34 Dong, X. and Ping, W. (2010). Study on the causes of hypertension with improved BP neural network. In: *2010 International Conference on E-Health Networking Digital Ecosystems and Technologies (EDT)*, 21–24. Shenzhen.

35 Oikawa, T., Obara, T., Ohkubo, T. et al. (2006). Characteristics of resistant hypertension determined by self-measured blood pressure at home and office blood pressure measurements: the J-HOME study. *Journal of Hypertension* 24 (9): 1737–1743.

36 Das, T., Guha, S., Banerjee, N., and Basak, P. (2017). Development of thermistor based low cost high sensitive respiration rate measurement system using audio software with audio input. In: *2017 Third International Conference on Biosignals, Images and Instrumentation (ICBSII)*, 1–3. Chennai.

37 Chen, Y., Zhang, H., and Wang, N. (2008). Body temperature monitor and alarm system used in hospital based on 1-wire and wireless communication technology. In: *2008 International Workshop on Education Technology and Training & 2008 International Workshop on Geoscience and Remote Sensing*, 401–404. Shanghai.

38 Fallah-Haghmohammadi, H. and Necsulecsu, D. (2017). Fever detection for dynamic human environment using sensor fusion. In: *2017 International Conference on Optimization of Electrical and Electronic Equipment (OPTIM) & 2017 Intl Aegean Conference on Electrical Machines and Power Electronics (ACEMP)*, 881–886. Brasov.

39 Shukla, R., Somani, S.B., and Shete, V.V. (2016). Wireless blood glucose monitoring system. In: *2016 International Conference on Inventive Computation Technologies (ICICT)*, 1–4. Coimbatore.

40 Eigner, G., Sas, P.I., and Kovács, L. (2014). Continuous glucose monitoring systems in the service of artificial pancreas. In: *2014 IEEE 9th IEEE International Symposium on Applied Computational Intelligence and Informatics (SACI)*, 117–122. Timisoara.

41 Larkai, D.L. and Wu, R. (2015). Wireless heart rate monitor in personal emergency response system. In: *2015 IEEE 18th International Symposium on Design and Diagnostics of Electronic Circuits & Systems*, 299–300. Belgrade.

42 Kioumars, A.H. and Tang, L. (2011). Wireless network for health monitoring: heart rate and temperature sensor. In: *2011 Fifth International Conference on Sensing Technology*, 362–369. Palmerston North.

43 Fan, Y.J., Yin, Y.H., Xu, L.D. et al. (2014). IoT-based smart rehabilitation system. *IEEE Transactions on Industrial Informatics* 10 (2): 1568–1577.

44 Ranannavare, L.B. and Suma (2020). IoT based rehabilitation system for patients and elderly people. *International Journal of Advanced Research in Computer Science* 11 (1): 236–240.

45 Buranapanichkit, D. et al. (2019). A patient monitoring system for multiple IoT rehabilitation devices. In: *2019 16th International Conference on*

Electrical Engineering/Electronics, Computer, Telecommunications and Information Technology (ECTI-CON), 834–837. Pattaya, Chonburi, Thailand.

46 Islam, S.M.R., Kwak, D., Kabir, M.H. et al. (2015). The internet of things for health care: a comprehensive survey. *IEEE Access* 3: 678–708.

47 Dohr, A., Modre-Opsrian, R., Drobics, M. et al. (2010). The Internet of Things for Ambient Assisted Living. In: *2010 Seventh International Conference on Information Technology: New Generations*, 804–809.

48 Zhang, X.M. and Zhang, N. (2011). An Open, Secure and Flexible Platform Based on Internet of Things and Cloud Computing for Ambient Aiding Living and Telemedicine. In: *2011 International Conference on Computer and Management (CAMAN)*, 1–4.

49 Pateraki, Maria, Fysarakis, Konstantinos, Sakkalis, Vangelis, Spanoudakis, George, Varlamis, Iraklis, Maniadakis, Michail, Lourakis, Manolis, Ioannidis, Sotiris, Cummins, Nicholas, Schuller, Björn, Loutsetis, Evangelos, Koutsouris, Dimitrios "Biosensors and Internet of Things in smart healthcare applications: challenges and opportunities", (2019).

50 Palmroth, A., Salpavaara, T., Vuoristo, P. et al. (2020). Materials and orthopedic applications for bioresorbable inductively coupled resonance sensors. *ACS Applied Materials & Interfaces* 12 (28): 31148–31161. https://doi.org/10.1021/acsami.0c07278.

51 Kilic, T., Valinhas, A.T.D.S., Wall, I. et al. (2018). Label-free detection of hypoxia-induced extracellular vesicle secretion from MCF-7 cells. *Scientific Reports* 8 (1) https://doi.org/10.1038/s41598-018-27203-9.

52 Economou, A., Karapetis, S., Nikoleli, G.P., Nikolelis, D., Bratakou, S., Varzakas, T. (2017). "Enzyme-based Sensors".

53 Kalra, S., Kumar, M.J., and Dhawan, A. (2020). Reconfigurable FET biosensor for a wide detection range and electrostatically tunable sensing response. *IEEE Sensors Journal* 20 (5): 2261–2269.

54 Gawali, D.H. and Wadhai, V.M. (2017). Technology innovations, challenges and emerging trends in wearable bio-sensor development. In: *2017 International Conference on Computing, Communication, Control and Automation (ICCUBEA)*, 1–6.

55 Pau, J.L., Núñez, C.G., Marín, A.G. et al. (2013). Metal oxide nanowires as building blocks for light detectors, gas sensors and biosensors. In: *2013 Spanish Conference on Electron Devices*, 171–174. Valladolid.

56 Jacobs, T., Gomide, A., Kahne, T. et al. (2007). Micro fluidic biosensor system based on quartz crystal resonators for fast online adherent cell proliferation and stimulation analysis. In: *Sensors, 2007 IEEE*, 720–723. Atlanta, GA.

6

A Review of e-Healthcare System of India and Thailand

Shanu Bhardwaj, S.N. Panda, Priyanka Datta, Rajesh Kumar Kaushal, and Naveen Kumar

Chitkara University Institute of Engineering and Technology, Chitkara University, Punjab, India

6.1 Introduction

e-health care is the technology that leads to quality treatment for patients, devices that improve the quality of life, and diagnostic tools for every human. e-health defines the use of various sensors that capture parameters of the human body. The doctors use the sensor data for the better treatment of the patients. The latest technology, i.e., Internet of Things (IoT), improves the health care system [1]. It is the intersection of the medical sensors, smartphones or tablets, and embedded devices to design a system that pro vides real-time healthcare to the patients, doctors, and medical caretakers to reduce time, save lives, and diminish expenses [2]. The concept of smart health must satisfy two main conditions. The first one is the achievement of better diagnostic tools and good treatment for patients. The second condition is recognized through the upgrading of life quality [3].

IoT is a platform where the sensors or devices or objects present in the network can communicate independently with other objects in the network [4]. It can send and receive data over the Internet without human interference. Nowadays people are becoming more concerned about health, but due to hectic workload or limitations due to aging, people are unable to visit a doctor personally at regular intervals, and thus this type of system is very helpful for them. The revolution in modern technologies such as IoT is reshaping the healthcare system with challenging socioeconomic and technological prospects [5].

IoT-Enabled Smart Healthcare Systems, Services and Applications, First Edition.
Edited by Shalli Rani, Maheswar Rajagopal, Neeraj Kumar and Syed Hassan Ahmed Shah.

In this chapter, we will study the latest technology used in Thailand and India for the last 10 years in the field of smart healthcare so that we can propose those technologies to other Southeast Asian underdeveloped countries for the better treatment of their citizens. In India, smart healthcare is gradually changing the way health services are delivered. Telemedicine and teleradiology, too, have emerged as potent tools to deliver healthcare in remote areas that lack local healthcare resources.

The remainder of the chapter is organized as follows: Section 6.2 describes the literature review of the e-healthcare system of India and Thailand. Section 6.3 presents the problem statement of the chapter. Section 6.4 illustrates the methodology used. Section 6.5 demonstrates the discussion section in which analysis result of each parameter is discussed. Finally, the conclusion section is presented.

6.2 Literature Review

6.2.1 India

Natarajan [6] presents a useful approach for e-health with the spirit to improve the e-healthcare system. The main objective of this approach is to attain the following schema in the e-healthcare system of India:

1) Enable simple sharing of organizational data.
2) Enable prominent access of information between dissimilar systems.
3) Enable cost effectiveness in e-healthcare.

Natarajan presents the problems that the current system faces and the solutions to tackle the problems. This paper works on the following parameters to enhance the e-Health care system:

1) Computerization of all healthcare data.
2) Computerization of e-health card.
3) Ease in the communication, i.e., smooth appointments with doctors.

Natarajan (2012) [7] solves health-related issues with the help of the latest technologies, the IoT. It also defines the architectural view of e-health or smart healthcare service, which was targeted to provide healthcare qualitatively to the citizens. By the use of this architectural view, the body parameters of patients can be measured in real time with the help of sensors. Sensors can collect the body parameters of the patient and the collected data is transferred to the Arduino Uno and then, further transfer the data to the cloud by making use of Wi-Fi modules. The information gathered was stored in a MySQL database. The database manages the data and provides access to that data. With the help of an Android application, the user or the patient can easily view the data.

Viswanathan et al. (2012) [8] present a study on telemedicine care in diabetes in rural areas. The Indian Council of Medical Research estimates that 62.5 million people suffer from diabetes. Moreover, there are many facilities provided to diabetic patients in urban areas, whereas 70% of the population lives in rural areas. This percentage was increased due to insufficient or lack of awareness, illiteracy, little access to healthcare due to problems in transportation, and lack of professionals in diabetes. The screening or checking for diabetes is hardly done in rural areas, which results in improper treatment. The research came up with a model of diabetes healthcare to care for patients in a more effective and affordable manner using a mobile vehicle or van having equipment for the treatment to diagnose, and in emergency cases, they can contact an expert with the help of trained technicians using satellite communication. In this paper, it was concluded that cost-effective healthcare can be achieved with telemedicine projects.

Raman et al. [9] study a telehealth program in the southern rural area of India. According to this paper, different teleservices were provided in the southern region of India. These teleservices were telepathology, telemedicine, telescreens, and many for remote treatment in the rural regions of southern India.

Srivastava et al. [10] present a secure model of e-health care in India. The survey of this paper describes that in urban areas, 75% of qualified and quality doctors' practices. Similarly, in the semi-urban area, only 23% and the rural area where the majority of the patient come is just 2%. And there is not any national insurance scheme for healthcare in India. Thus, in this paper, the model is enabled with the cloud to track and maintain the record of patients remotely for the treatment in rural as well as in urban areas.

Karthikeyan et al. (2015) [11] provide information about the service of emergency healthcare in India. According to this paper, healthcare professionals say that due to the lack of communication between patients and healthcare staff, there was a gap in providing healthcare to the patients in case of emergencies. So the conclusion was, there would be "on-demand software services" by which the patient can be treated remotely by the doctor by generating the information in the cloud.

Natarajan et al. [7] describe an efficient exchange of medical information with the help of the IoT, which has been shown to be helpful for the patients as well as doctors. According to this paper, the research done by all other researchers were:

1) A platform of Health-IoT, which is based on the collection of Packaging, BioSensor, and smart medicine box; and
2) RFID technology, which is used for healthcare in IoT.

This research shows the applications of IoT in informational industrial sectors such as healthcare services. However, IoT provides heterogeneous solutions to the problems. In the paper, an efficient and effective communication from one machine to another machine was gained for smart healthcare.

Ghamari et al. [12]. In this survey paper, the current progression of wearable and smart health monitoring technology has strong prospects to change the future of the smart healthcare system by enabling the remote monitoring of patients. This health monitoring system consists of wearable sensors that monitor the physiological parameters of the patient. The data collected by the sensors were received by using the wireless communicational protocol (WBANs). The main aim of this survey was to remotely monitor the elderly or ill patients in their own residential places.

Kumar and Ahmad [13] define the use of telemedicine and e-health services in India for public health. According to this paper, there is a great difference in quality and in access to healthcare in rural and urban areas. The availability of healthcare services in India was so small that it was bonded to the following activities:

1) Medical transcriptions;
2) Telemedicine;
3) Customer service through the Internet; and
4) Awareness with the help of portals.

Catarinucci et al. [14] define a smart architecture for smart monitoring as well as tracking of patients and biomedical devices in hospitals and in any medical institutes. A smart hospital system (SHS) depends on heterogeneous technologies, and the technologies used were RFID, wireless sensor network (WSN), and mobile devices. The SHS is capable of collecting real-time parameters of the patient with the help of a ultra-low-power hybrid sensing network (HSN). The data obtained with the help of sensors are delivered to the main centers where the advanced monitoring makes the system accessible by rural as well as remote users via web service.

Kaur and Jasuja (2017) [4] propose a remote health monitoring system based on IoT, bearing low cost and low power. The system makes use of temperature and pulse rate sensor along with Arduino Uno and Blynk.

The body temperature and pulse rate of a person sensed by the sensors are sent to the cloud with the help of an Ethernet shield and are displayed on the Blynk mobile application preinstalled on the android phone or iOS. The system is very useful and valuable to the society especially for the senior citizens since they can have a regular checkup sitting at their homes.

Ila Sehrawat (2017) [15]. The objective of this paper is to find the gaps and barriers that were hidden in the expansion of m-health services in India. This paper helps to remove the two crucial problems concerned with healthcare: lack of communication and the distance between doctor and patient in the urban to rural areas.

There are a few useful mobile applications and websites that were developed for the self-monitoring system to overcome the above two crucial problems:

1) M Health Basic: It is the website that provides thorough information about health on mobile in India.
2) OB Insulin: It is the mobile application that helps to determine the initial dose of a drug (insulin) for pregnant women.
3) Health PIE (Patient Information and Empowerment system): It is the mobile application that helps to maintain personal information, scheduling of treatment, statistics of personalized health, doctor on just one call, and many more items.
4) Mswasthya CDAC (Centre for Development of Advanced Computing, India): It is the mobile application that helps in monitoring the patient's blood pressure, diabetes, calorie counting, calculating BMI, searching doctors, emergencies, provides facts for nutrition, OPD schedule, and alerts for vaccination.
5) HealthCare atHome: It is the website that provides high standard clinic care and treatment protocols to patients.
6) Healthy You Card: It is the mobile application that provides a search engine to search for the doctors, hospitals, centers for diagnostic, booking of appointments online, SMS, and e-mail facility for updating and reminders about appointments.
7) Lybrate: It is a mobile application that provides emergency facility to patients by just one click, booking of appointments, and also helps in maintaining medical records of the patients.

Jamali [11] provides a comparative analysis of the mobile healthcare system in rural and urban India. According to this paper, a WSN is a powerful tool for collecting medical-related data in healthcare situations in rural as well as urban areas. The network sensors were used mainly in urban areas.

The sensors were used to collect the data and transmit the information remotely to the health professional.

Patil and Suralkar (2018) [16]. The aim of this paper is to transmit the monitoring parameters of the patient with the help of wireless network sensors. The IoT method is adapted for accessing patient's parameters remotely as well as in the local area. In the paper, heart rate, body temperature, and respiration rate can be monitored with a Raspberry Pi. When the Internet is connected to the board of the Raspberry Pi, it will act as a server. Then, this server automatically sends the data to the main or web server. With the help of this server, the parameters of the patient are monitored with the help of a web page, and these can be monitored anytime, anywhere, all over the world, using laptops, tablets, and smartphones.

Kaur and Sharma (2018) [17] present a review of the research literature on telemedicine services. Telemedicine provides a platform to communicate and exchange data between doctors and patients over the high-speed Internet. It is useful for providing consultation through videoconferencing to patients residing in remote areas. The present study is an attempt to access the efforts made by the researchers in the fields of telemedicine services in India.

Kaur et al. [18] is a review paper on telemedicine services in India. It explores various emerging trends in telemedicine and elaborate associated issues. Different mobile apps have launched for of telemedicine:

1) Vaccine Tracker was launched in April 2016 to help the parents to track the immunization of their children and helps them ensuring complete and timely vaccinations.
2) India Fights Dengue was launched in April 2016 and enables the users to check dengue symptoms and get the nearest hospital and blood bank information and even shares feedback.
3) NHP (National Health Portal, India) Swasth Bharat was launched in April 2016. It is an NHP Directory Service (provides information supplied by hospitals across India).
4) Pradhan Mantri Surakshit Matritva Abhiyan mobile app launched in November 2016. This application reports information related to pregnancy across different states.
5) Mera Aspataal mobile application was launched in August 2016 and provides information related to pregnancy.

Elhoseny et al. [19] improve the secure transmission of medical data from the patient's residence to the doctor in the hospital. This model is based on the integration of steganography techniques and a hybrid encryption strategy to make the transmission vastly secured in e-Healthcare services. Data transmission plays a very significant role in the e-healthcare system. This research paper presents a security hybrid model providing security to the medical text information in images. This encryption schema is basically built for using the combinations of Advanced Encryption Standards (AES) and several algorithms: Adleman, Rivest, and Shamir. This model was started by encrypting the data that is secret and then hides the conclusion in the cover image by using 2D/DWT/1L and 2D/DWT/2L (DWT stands for discrete wavelet transform).

6.2.2 Thailand

Phabphal and Hirunpatch [20] designed a method by utilizing a mobile network in teleradiology consultation done by neurologists. Doctors can assist outdoor patients, those who are away from the hospital and are suspected of having a stroke. In Thailand there is a very limited number of neurologist specialists, so the author had proposed the device that can assist patients with minimum cost. The system was designed on a PC to send images, and a PDA or phone will receive it. The author has done it with good accuracy, but the cases that have been studied are very few.

Kijsanayotin et al. (2008) [21] improve the UTAUT (unified theory of acceptance and use of technology) structural model for understanding the factors that prevent community health centers from adopting health IT in Thailand and also validate the model of IT adoption in the context of healthcare of the country. A research design was used for studying community health centers' (CHCs') IT use and adoption. The researchers used a randomly collected sample of 1607 stratified regionally CHCs among 9806 CHCs. This data was collected using a cross-sectional survey (a self-administered questionnaire), which had a response rate of 82%. The proposed model had used partial least squares (PLS) modeling. The result of the developed model showed that the level of IT acceptance was high among CHCs staff. The resulting analysis recommended that acceptance of IT influenced effort expectancy, performance expectancy, voluntariness, and social influence. This study showed that CHCs staff had adopted health IT in Thailand. This result implicates that both health informatics research and health IT was developing in Thailand. It had also explained that modeling of the PLS path had worked well in the field study and in the complex model used for exploratory research purposes.

Jaranit et al. (2010) [22] propose a module that can effectively improve the immunization and antenatal care for those who are living in the border area in Thailand, as they are underserved. The web-based mobile technology had been used for developing the module. The proposed module had been successfully integrated into remote rural areas. The author's module can be further expanded on other diseases also.

Meankaew et al. (2010) [23] propose a repetitive malaria control and prevention program for improving the supervision of malaria cases among an underserved population of Thailand. This research paper designed a device integrating mobile and web-based technology for replacing the existing paper-based and manual activities used by healthcare staff for providing treatment to the malaria-affected villagers. When a patient was detected and registered into the system, treatment details and case investigation were stored into the database. Checkup was scheduled, and the status of the patient was uploaded when the healthcare staff visited the patient's home for routine checkups using a cell phone. This module can generate graphical messages and text for abstract detail of malaria and its statistics, which can be automatically sent to the predetermined malaria specialists for analyzing the situation. The patient's data were stored securely so that only the person who had the privilege to access the data can access.

Ampornpunt [24] studied the scenario of IT on Thai hospitals and proposed a model for IT organizational adoption that includes vital hospital characteristics and facilitating management. This paper had estimated the acceptance of computerized physician order entry (CPOE) and electronic medical records (EMR). This study allowed other subsequent studies to track the use of IT by Thai hospitals.

Vanessa et al. (2012) [25] provide an effort to solve issues and improve the rural healthcare system using mobile technology. They have significantly contributed to the emerging field of the healthcare system in rural areas in Thailand and other Asian countries for the use of tablets or PC, based on the TCM (technology-community-management) model. It was found that community factors such as training, needs, and ownership are crucial in the usage of the Family Folder Collector (FFC).

Montri Wiboonrat (2012) [26]. The aim of this paper is to support the emergency medical services (EMS) staff at the remote location of Bangkok by combining online EMR for providing patients' data on hot-spot so that the staff of EMS can consult a physician and get an appropriate decision. Treatment quality and cost efficiency were accomplished by an ecosystem of combining insurance policies, Medicare, tactical patient's data, EMR, EMS, telematics support, vital signs, and teleconferencing from the emergency spot. This paper proposes the model for e-EMS online services along with vital requirements and essentially combined ecosystem of software, hardware, data communication, and architecture of a networking system that was supported by EMR and EMS system. This proposed model can be used as a foundation for integrating EMR and e-EMS system development, which will increase the response speed to medical diagnoses and privacy, treatment, security, safety, and maintaining the privacy of patients' data, reliability, and availability of doctors 24/7 for supporting emergency departments (EDs).

Pasierb (2013) [27]. According to the author the healthcare system is knowledge-based and depends mainly on activities for improving quality services. The future scope is to pay attention to enabling knowledge transfer based on ICT by minimizing financial and organizational obstacles. In this paper, eHealth services aimed at grid-based applications and technologies related to geographic information systems work with location-based services.

Chen et al. [28] propose a conceptual framework on privacy for mHealth. It can be used for itemized properties based on privacy. Many challenges were identified; work needs to be done on it immediately since the health care system is spreading rapidly.

Namahoot and Brueckner [29]. The authors explore the usage of telemedicine for unhealthy people living in rural areas of Thailand. They had proposed a system, TEDIST (Telemedicine Diagnosis System for Rural Thailand), through which people can consult the community health center for treatment from their mobile phones. TEDIST stands for Telemedicine Diagnosis System for Rural Thailand. TEDIST consists of three levels: clients, an application server, and a DBMS. The database server used for these purposes was MySQL Server 4.0. The limitation of the system was that they consulted limited patients and only presented few conditions in their system.

Wacharasint [30]. This author implemented the Tele-ICU idea for people in rural areas who were living far away from hospitals in urban areas. The proposed device helped junior doctors and nurses who were present at rural health center ICUs to consult senior as well as specialist doctors from urban areas, through audio, video, or teleconferencing using a free application such as Skype and LINE for providing better treatment to their patients. Though its implementation is challenging, in the future it can be used by middle- to low-income countries.

Boonchieng et al. [31]. The aim of this paper was to study location services of GPS, which are available on almost every mobile device along with health systems of the district and saving data on a private cloud system. The mobile application is developed for iOS, web-based platforms, and Android. This system had two parts of district health data: a form for individual health-related data and forms for recording resident data, which were approved and developed by sharing public opinion and hearing. A web-based application was developed using PHP, HTML5, and MySQL for managing database systems. The proposed software can display information in varieties of views from old-style tables to different types of layered graphics, high resolution and incorporated map-related location data with views of the street from Google maps. Capabilities such as multi-extension exporting are also given, utilizing a platform such as PNG, JPG, PDF, and XLS. The collection of data was from March 2013 to March 2014. The data was collected by heath volunteers and youth volunteers who had successfully completed the application training. The generated report by the system has a major advantage for the district hospital of Saraphi: this data can be further used by the healthcare providers for providing healthcare services at patients' homes and can also promote activities regarding healthcare that can benefit people of the community.

Jantavongso [32] explains the role of eHealth, also known as ICT, in health and social media. As eHealth in Thailand is flourishing rapidly, it becomes crucial to maintain patients' data confidentially and security. The author proposes a research cycle of three stages: building of theory, testing the theory, and refinement of the theory, using digital technologies and the Internet.

Wongwai et al. [33] propose a cost-effective system that can store and forward telemedicine for ROP (retinopathy of prematurity) for high-risk infants by using analytical decision models. They also use one-way and probabilistic sensitivity analysis for considering the uncertainty parameter.

Kato et al. [34]. The authors develop an eHealth system that is based on semantic and ontology web technologies. For implementing user interfaces they use JSP and server technologies because it helps to execute Java programs that activate Thai herbal references. To run servlet and JSP, a Tomcat application server is used. A MySQL database is used to store static information. This can derive information of Thai herbs for treatments based on the real-life knowledge about traditional Thai herbal medication, which is symptom-based treatment.

Victoria and Vanessa (2015) [35]. This paper examines the global impact of ICT in health through the use of mobile devices, basically targeting children and women of the rural and remote regions of developing countries. The systematic research for this paper contains qualitative and quantitative studies published in 2002, 2009, 2010, and 2011. At this time, the majority of these initiatives are at the initial stage, and the literature survey and publication on this topic are growing.

Narattharaksa et al. [36, 37] investigate the data that healthcare personnel of Thailand think are important for successfully running EMR systems.

These factors can help managers, stakeholders, and administrators of the public e-healthcare system. The advantage of this research paper is that it covers a huge number of random samples of healthcare workers, mostly doctors and nurses, who use the system.

Zaman et al. [38] predict the existing and upcoming scope of eHealth in the field of healthcare support system. The newly developed eHealth system can play a crucial role in remote places of developing and emerging countries though it seems problematic due to the absence of communication infrastructure. e-health was a challenging field for providing benefits to public health if it was combined with the traditional medical system. More systematic strategies are required for the evaluation, development, and planning of eHealth. National and international organizations should emphasize the betterment of eHealth technology so that it is successfully adopted by societies for patients' benefits. Moreover, mHealth should not be taken as the ultimate solution for increasing the exposure of healthcare distribution. It should work in parallel with traditional clinical visits and routine checkups. Lastly, new and upcoming eHealth technologies have a huge possibility to remove the gaps between the healthcare provider and patients. Integrating technologies into the healthcare system can improve patient-oriented healthcare systems.

Pal et al. [39]. The objective of this paper is to examine the main factors that affect the elderly users from accepting the smart healthcare system. Many thread factors are identified from which a risk model can be created. This model can help stakeholders define better policies that will ensure success in the field of the smart healthcare system.

Kamolphiwong et al. (2018) [40] investigate the effects of packet delay and packet loss variations, particularly for lungs and heart sounds with the sound of auscultations in real-time services over the Internet. They find that both sounds are most sensitive to packet delay than packet loss. Heart sounds are less sensitive than lungs sounds because of timing interpretation; a prototype of tele-auscultation in real time has been developed, which tries to minimize the variation in packet delay. They also find that the visualization of the waveform of auscultations in real time can help in increasing the doctor's confidence level by interpreting sound. In their study, tele-auscultation has been summarized into three compositions: client application, stethoscope, and application server. The processes were defined as collecting information, processing, transmission, and then display. Some more techniques are suggested for improving the quality of services, e.g., user interfaces and noise reduction.

6.3 Problem Statement

A review of e-healthcare in India and Thailand is a comparative study of smart health in both countries. The governments of both countries is launching many new schemes regarding healthcare, such as Ayushman Bharat-National Health Protection Mission, which are suitable to the community in order to meet the healthcare facilities. One such problem is that the people living in rural areas are not able to make use of such schemes. So this study is conducted in order to achieve all the objectives to provide the resources to the people living in rural areas too, with the use of the latest technologies. Therefore, an attempt will be made by the researchers to conduct a comparative study between both countries, India and Thailand, on the basis of e-healthcare to improve the status of the health system in each and every region of both countries.

6.4 Methodology

The present comparative study is accomplished by collecting published empirical data related to e-healthcare of two cross-Asian countries, India and Thailand. This review was carried out in June 2018. The literature of the last 10 years, from 2008 to 2018, is reviewed. The related literature is searched through various combinations of descriptors such as "IoT and eHealth," "smart healthcare system," and "healthcare" on popular search engines such as Google Scholar, Science-Direct, and CiteSeerX. A total of 54 research papers have reviewed e-healthcare in India and Thailand. After exclusion, 42 research papers are included in the study. The 12 research papers are excluded because the data provided is not relevant according to the review criteria. This paper focuses on the three main parameters that are the rural area, cost effectiveness, and technology.

6.5 Discussion

6.5.1 Country Differences

This review paper includes a comparative study about the healthcare system in two Asian countries, India and Thailand (Figure 6.1). In India, e-healthcare is improving, but still, there are some issues that need to be revolved, same as for Thailand. In both countries, a majority of citizens resides in rural areas whereas the constraint of healthcare system in this

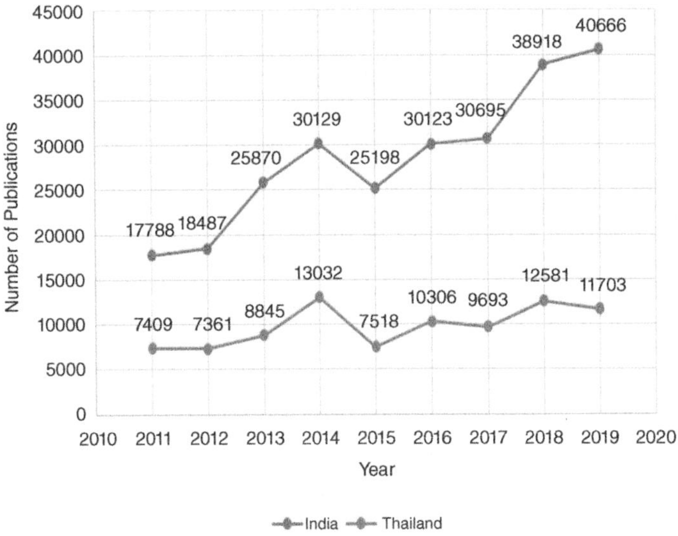

Figure 6.1 Number of publications of India and Thailand on e healthcare system.

arena is not worthy. The technologies used by India for the development of an e-healthcare system are less expensive than the ones used by Thailand. Thailand is more advanced than India in its healthcare system.

6.5.2 Parameters Considered

6.5.2.1 Rural Area

This review paper includes data of 30 research papers out of which the number of papers focused to improve the healthcare system by prefix letter "e," i.e., E-healthcare. Both countries pay much attention to the rural area because the people living there don't get proper healthcare services and suffer a lot (see Table 6.1 and Figure 6.2). This is the reason there is a bond between e-health and rural area. In India, patients in the rural areas have to visit the doctors for treatments who are far away from them, but in the case of Thailand, the patients in the rural areas have the means to get treated at their place. To overcome this problem, researchers have proposed different systems that solve their problems remotely to an extent.

6.5.2.2 Technology

Both countries are using different technologies for the improvement of their e-healthcare systems (Figure 6.3). In most research papers of India, the technology cloud has been used for storing the patient data securely,

Table 6.1 Difference between health facilities in rural and urban India [41].

S. No.	Predictable	Rural area (per 1000 person)	Urban area (per 1000 person)
1.	Qualified doctors	0.6	3.4
2.	Hospital beds	0.2	3.0
3.	Infant mortality rate	0.074	0.044
4.	Births attended by doctors	33.5%	73.3%

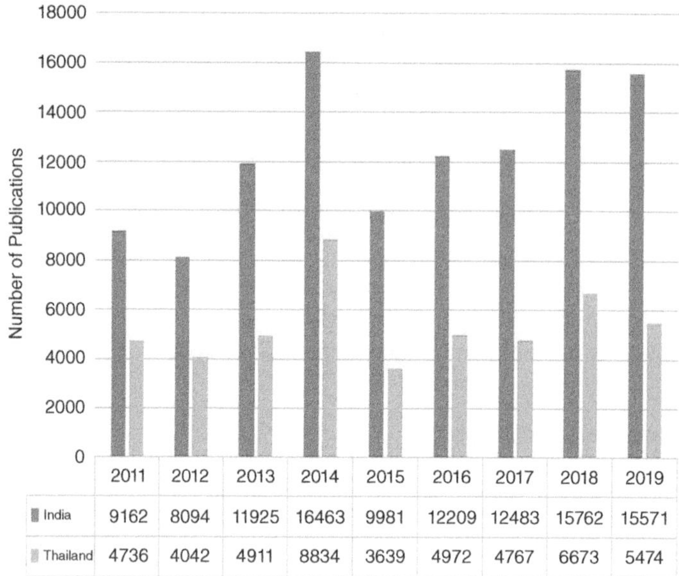

Figure 6.2 Number of publication on rural e-healthcare system in India and Thailand.

whereas, in the papers of Thailand, the concept of EMR for storing patients data and maintaining the privacy is used. The microcontroller used in the smart healthcare system in India is Raspberry Pi and Arduino Uno; on the other hand, Thailand makes use of Arduino 1.6.7 IDE.

The telemedicine [42] concept is used by both countries, but Thailand also uses advanced systems such as teleICU, tele-pathology, tele-psychiatry, tele-radiology, and tele-dermatology. This advanced system requires high-speed Internet, which is available in Thailand, as 23.9 million are active users of the Internet. In India, sensors used for the smart healthcare system

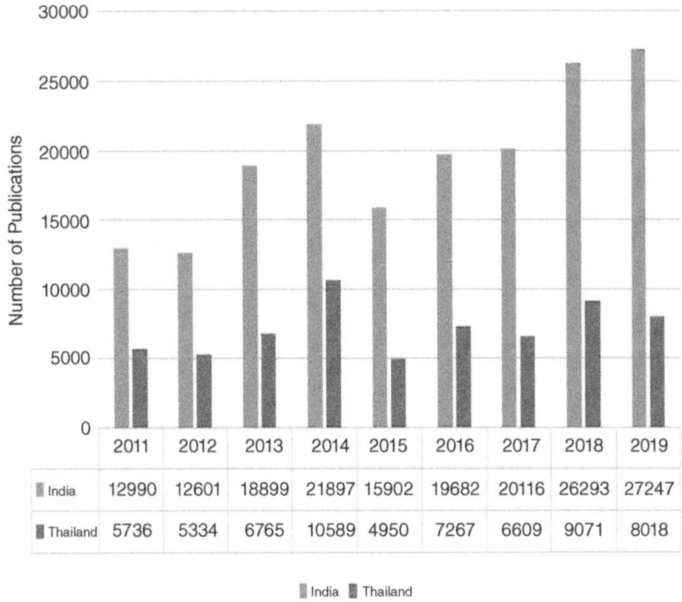

	2011	2012	2013	2014	2015	2016	2017	2018	2019
India	12990	12601	18899	21897	15902	19682	20116	26293	27247
Thailand	5736	5334	6765	10589	4950	7267	6609	9071	8018

Figure 6.3 Number of publication on technology used in e-healthcare system of India and Thailand.

are temperature wireless sensors, heart rate detection sensors, and pulse rate sensors, while in Thailand, the sensors used are the bio-medical sensors, which are a combination of temperature, heart rate, and pulse sensors. Thus, it can be concluded that Thailand is technologically more advanced than India.

6.5.2.3 Cost-Effectiveness

The third parameter that we have considered while writing this chapter is cost effectiveness. The conclusion is that the technologies used for the smart healthcare system in India are less expensive with respect to Thailand. Consequently, the publication rate on cost effectiveness of the e-healthcare system in India is more than Thailand as shown in Figure 6.4.

6.6 Conclusion

This chapter provides a comprehensive analysis of the research work carried out in the field of e-healthcare in India and Thailand for the last 10 years. The analysis concludes that the number of publications is higher

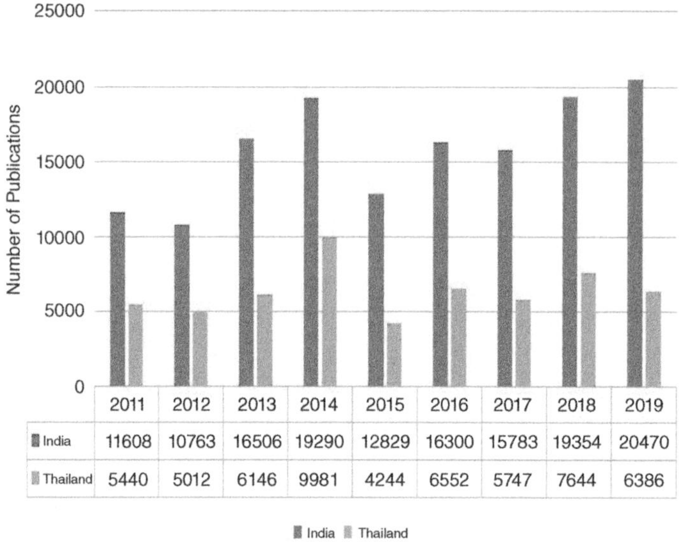

Figure 6.4 Number of publication on cost-effectiveness of e-healthcare system in India and Thailand.

in India as compared to Thailand. The comparison between the nations is done by three parameters, namely, rural area, technology, and cost effectiveness. These are the most relevant parameters in the field of healthcare since much work has not been done yet in this era. There are still more parameters that could be considered to improve the e-healthcare system of both countries. Future work includes uncovering other parameters that have not yet been studied.

References

1 Dinesh, K., Vijayalakshmi, K., Nirosha, C., and Krishna, I.S.R. (2018). IoT based smart health care monitoring system. *International Journal of Institutional and Industrial Research* 3 (1): 22–24.

2 Chandrashekar, R., Padma, R., & Hemalatha, G. Analysis and Performance Of E-Health Iot-Enabled Healthcare Solutions With Using Integrated Fog And Cloud.

3 Agrawal, S. and Vieira, D. (2013). A survey on internet of things. *Abakós* 1 (2): 78–95.

4 Bhardwaj, S. and Panda, S.N. (2019). SDWSN: software-defined wireless sensor network. *JITEE* 8 (12): 1064–1071.

5 Islam, S.M.R., Kwak, D., Kabir, H. et al. (2015). The internet of things for health care: a comprehensive survey. *IEEE Access* 3: 678–708.

6 Natarajan, M. (2015). Impact of information technology to e-health strategies with special reference to India. *Asian Journal of Library and Information Science* 2 (1–4): 26–35.

7 Natarajan, K., Prasath, B., and Kokila, P. (2016). Smart health care system using internet of things. *Journal of Network Communications and Emerging Technologies* 6 (3): 37–42.

8 Mohan, V. and Pradeepa, R. (2014). Telemedicine in diabetes care: in rural India, a new prevention project seeks to fill in the screening gap. *IEEE Pulse* 5 (3): 22–25.

9 Raman, R. et al. (2005). Telehealth program for diabetic retinopathy in rural South India: a pilot study. *eHealth International*: 13–18.

10 Srivastava, S., Pane, N.A.M., and Abraham, A. (2013). A secured model for Indian EHealth system A. Security and privacy in "Aadhaar" "Aadhaar". In: *Ehealth Services International Conference on Information Assurance and Security (IAS)*, 96–101.

11 Jamali, M.C. (2017). A comparative analysis upon Mobile healthcare system and services: a case study of rural India. *Journal of Emergency Medicine and Critical Care* 3 (1): 1–4.

12 Ghamari, M., Janko, B., Sherratt, R.S. et al. (2016). A survey on wireless body area networks for ehealthcare systems in residential environments. *Sensors (Switzerland)* 16 (6): 1–33.

13 Kumar, A. and Ahmad, S. (2015). A review study on utilization of telemedicine and e-health services in public health. *Asian Pacific Journal of Health Sciences* 2: 60–68.

14 Catarinucci, L., De Donno, D., Mainetti, L. et al. (2015). An IoT-aware architecture for smart healthcare systems. *IEEE Internet of Things Journal* 2 (6): 515–526.

15 Bishnoi, N. and Sehrawat, A. (2013). Cloud computing architecture to aid telemedicine. *International Journal of Computer Science Engineering and Information Technology Research (IJCSEITR)* ISSN 2249-6831 3 (4): 13–18.

16 Gladies, E. J., & Abinaya, R. Supervising Physical Condition for Pernatal Ladies. Special Issue in Communication and Information Technology, 63.

17 Bensalah, M., Elouadi, A., and Mharzi, H. (2018). Integrating BIM in railway projects review & perspectives for Morocco and MENA. *International Journal of Recent Scientific Research* 9: 23398–23403.

18 Kuar, G., Kaur, P.P., Mal, M., and College, M. A review on telemedicine services in India. *International Journal of Advanced in Management, Technology and Engineering Sciences* 8 (1): 214–218.

19 Elhoseny, M., Ramírez-González, G., Abu-Elnasr, O.M. et al. (2018). Secure medical data transmission model for IoT-based healthcare systems. *IEEE Access* 6: 20596–20608.

20 Phabphal, K. and Hirunpatch, S. (2008). The effectiveness of low-cost teleconsultation for emergency head computer tomography in patients with suspected stroke. *Journal of Telemedicine and Telecare* 14 (8): 439–442.

21 Bhardwaj, S. and Panda, S.N. (2020). A roadmap of challenges for OpenFlow-SDN based IoT networks. *International Journal of Advanced Science and Technology* 29 (05): 947–961. Retrieved from http://sersc.org/journals/index.php/IJAST/article/view/9737.

22 Kaewkungwal, J., Singhasivanon, P., Khamsiriwatchara, A. et al. (2010). Application of smart phone in "Better Border Healthcare Program": a module for mother and child care. *BMC Medical Informatics and Decision Making* 10 (1): 69.

23 Ariani, A., Koesoema, A.P., and Soegijoko, S. (2017). Innovative healthcare applications of ICT for developing countries. In: *Innovative Healthcare Systems for the 21st Century*, 15–70. Cham: Springer.

24 Theera-Ampornpunt, N. (2011). Thai hospitals' adoption of information technology: a theory development and nationwide survey.

25 Chong, V.W.T., Lim, M.H., & Rodricks, R.M. (2012). Adoption, usage and impact of Family Folder Collector (FFC) on a mobile Android tablet device in rural Thailand.

26 Bhardwaj, S., Panda, S.N., and Datta, P. (2020). Comparison and performance evaluation of software-defined networking controllers. In: *2020 International Conference on Emerging Smart Computing and Informatics (ESCI)*, 276–281. IEEE.

27 Xu, L., Chen, G., Cao, J. et al. (2015). Optimizing energy efficiency for minimum latency broadcast in low-duty-cycle sensor networks. *ACM Transactions on Sensor Networks (TOSN)* 11 (4): 1–31.

28 Chen, H., Vasardani, M., & Winter, S. (2017). Geo-referencing place from everyday natural language descriptions. arXiv preprint arXiv:1710.03346.

29 Namahoot, C.S. and Brueckner, M. (2013). Tele-diagnosis system for rural Thailand. *International Scholarly and Scientific Research & Innovation* 7 (6).

30 Wacharasint, P. (2014). The role of health information technology on critical care services in Thailand. *Journal of the Medical Association of Thailand* 97 (1): 127–131.

31 Boonchieng, E., Boonchieng, W., Senaratana, W., and Singkaew, J. (2014). Development of mHealth for public health information collection, with GIS, using private cloud: a case study of Saraphi district, Chiang Mai,

Thailand. In: *2014 International Computer Science and Engineering Conference (ICSEC)*, 350–353. IEEE.

32 Jantavongso, S. (2015). Ethics, social media and e-health in Thailand. *Journal of the Thai Medical Informatics Association* 1 (1).

33 Wongwai, P., Kingkaew, P., Asawaphureekorn, S., and Kolatat, T. (2015). A store-and-forward telemedicine for retinopathy of prematurity screen: is it cost-effective in Thailand? *Asian Biomedicine* 9 (5): 665–673.

34 Kato, T., Maneerat, N., Varakulsiripunth, R. et al. (2009). Ontology-based E-health system with Thai herb recommendation. In: *Proceeding of the 6th International Joint Conference on Computer Science and Software Engineering (JCSSE2009)*, 172–177.

35 Victoria, V., & Nicogossian, A. (2011). mHealth: Saving lives with mobile technology.

36 Benyakorn, S. (2016). Implementing telepsychiatry in Thailand benefits and challenges. *Journal of the Medical Association of Thailand* 99: S260–S266.

37 Narattharaksa, K., Speece, M., Newton, C., and Bulyalert, D. (2016). Key success factors behind electronic medical record adoption in Thailand. *Journal of Health Organization and Management.*

38 Zaman, S.B., Hossain, N., Ahammed, S., and Ahmed, Z. (2017). Contexts and opportunities of e-health technology in medical care. *Journal of Medical Research and Innovation* 1 (2): AV1–AV4.

39 Pal, D., Funilkul, S., Charoenkitkarn, N., and Kanthamanon, P. (2018). Internet-of-things and smart homes for elderly healthcare: an end user perspective. *IEEE Access* 6: 10483–10496.

40 Ghuman, B.S. and Mehta, A. (2009). Health care services in India: problems and prospects. In: *International Conference on the Asian Social Protection in Comparative Perspective*, 7–9. Singapore: National University of singapore.

41 Bhardwaj, S. and Panda, S.N. (2020). A study on noninvasive body wearable sensors. In: *Intelligent Communication, Control and Devices*, 345–351. Singapore: Springer.

42 Kamolphiwong, S., Kamolphiwong, T., Saechow, S., and Chandeeying, V. (2018). *Real-Time Tele-Auscultation Consultation Services over the Internet: Effects of the Internet Quality of Service*, 139. eHealth: Making Health Care Smarter.

7

WSN- and IoT-Based Smart Surveillance Systems for Patients with Closed-Loop Alarm

Amit Sundas[1], Sumit Badotra[2], Shalli Rani[3], and Chhabildas Madhukar Gajare[1]

[1] *School of Engineering, Ajeenkya DY Patil University, Pune, India*
[2] *School of Computer Science & Engineering, Faculty of Engineering & Technology, Jain University, Karnataka, India*
[3] *Chitkara University Institute of Engineering and Technology, Chitkara University, Punjab, India*

7.1 Introduction

IoT is an extremely large network; it contains and consists of each electronic device such as mobile phones and home phones, connected home appliances, connected vehicles, and many more smart electronic objects. IoT has emerged as one of the most important technologies of the 21st century. IoT is now being used in every research area, security system, health science, or manufacturing of any objects or devices[1]. In short, we can say that IoT has made our daily life more reliable and easier. The most important features of IoT include receiving, storing, sending, and accessing different sensor data in real time from anywhere. The sensors are basically used to collect the information, such as time, temperature, humidity, body mass index (BMI), acceleration, and many more depending on the different kinds of sensors [2]. The sensor receives and stores information in real time and then sends that information to the cloud by using any kind of Wi-Fi module such as D1 mini NodeMCU, ESP8266 NodeMCU, or Bluetooth modules HC-05, with the help of a microprocessor or microcontroller.

IoT-Enabled Smart Healthcare Systems, Services and Applications, First Edition.
Edited by Shalli Rani, Maheswar Rajagopal, Neeraj Kumar and Syed Hassan Ahmed Shah.

7.1.1 Working of IoT

The working of the entire IoT process depends on its devices, such as smart watches, smartphones, Internet-connected washing machines, Internet-connected TVs, and many other electronic appliances; all these devices help each other to communicate with the IoT platform, which is shown in Figure 7.1 [3]. Further, the working of the entire IoT system depends on the following four fundamental components:

- **Devices or sensors:** In IoT, devices or sensors are the main components, which help us to collect data in real time from various environments. Data complexity depend upon their nature, whether it is an audio/video feed or a simple humidity-monitoring sensor. Many sensors consist of a single device, but they can perform multiple jobs. For example, a computer is a device consisting of multiple sensors in it, such as a camera, touchpad, and GPS, but it cannot sense these things [4].
- **Connectivity:** All the data collected from various devices or sensors is sent to a cloud platform. Further, to send the data to the cloud, the device needs to be connected through a communications medium. The mediums could be Wi-Fi, satellite, or mobile networks, WAN, Bluetooth, or Infrared [2–3].
- **Data or information processing:** Once the data is collected from the sensor, it is sent to the cloud, and then software performs the processing of the data. This whole process checking from taking humidity,

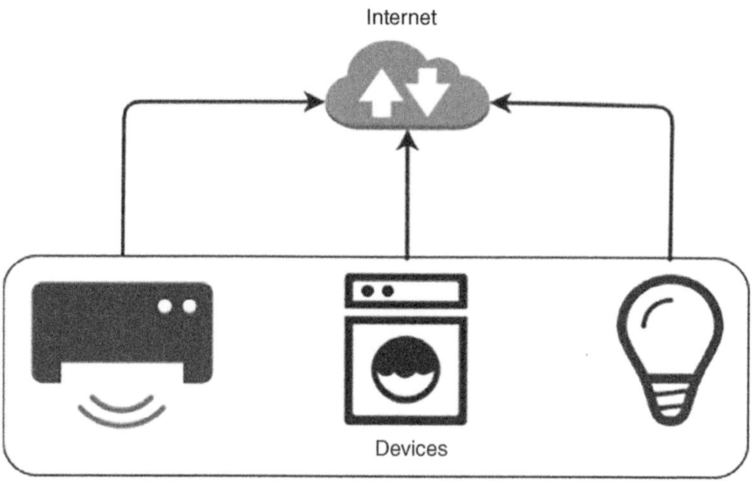

Figure 7.1 Working of IoT.

temperature readings from the devices like heaters or AC. Even so, sometimes it can get complex, such as identifying motion of objects on videos using computer vision [5].

- **User interface:** The data or information needs to be visible to the end user, for further operation. The data can be shown in terms of trigger alarms or by sending a text or email notification on their phones. In some cases, the user requires an IoT-based system interface, which is continuously monitoring and active. For example, a doctor wants to monitor patients from a remote location. If she wants to access the vital signs information of the patients, she can fetch this data in her phone using an application or web-based portal [4].

However, in some cases it can be two-way communication; basically, it all depends on the IoT system or application we are using. In this case, the user performs a task or action in a similar way, so the system also wants to perform the action, which can create a cascading effect. Put another way, the user only gives instructions to the device or system to perform that instruction. The device receives the commands and performs the task and gives output according to the instruction.

However, in some cases, it may also be two-way communication; basically, it depends on the IoT system or the application we use or want. In this case, the user does a task or action in the same way that the system also wants to do the action, which can create a cascading effect. Put another way, the user only gives instruction to the device or system to perform that instruction. The device receives the controls and performs their task and delivers the output as instructed.

7.1.2 Wireless Sensor Networks (WSNs)

As IoT surged as a prominent technology, the use of wireless sensor networks (WSNs) has grown rapidly. WSNs are webs of objects or devices that exchange data or information collected from the system field or a monitored ground via an over-the-air network [6]. The processed information is redirected via various nodes of the network, and with a gateway, the processed information or data is linked by each node to other networks such as a Wi-Fi network, also known as Wireless Ethernet.

A WSN is a wireless, or Wi-Fi-based, network that comprises a root, or base station, where the data is collected and organized (center location), and several wireless sensors. WSNs are used to continuously monitor and record emotional and physical environmental conditions and then send the collected information to the base station [7]. They

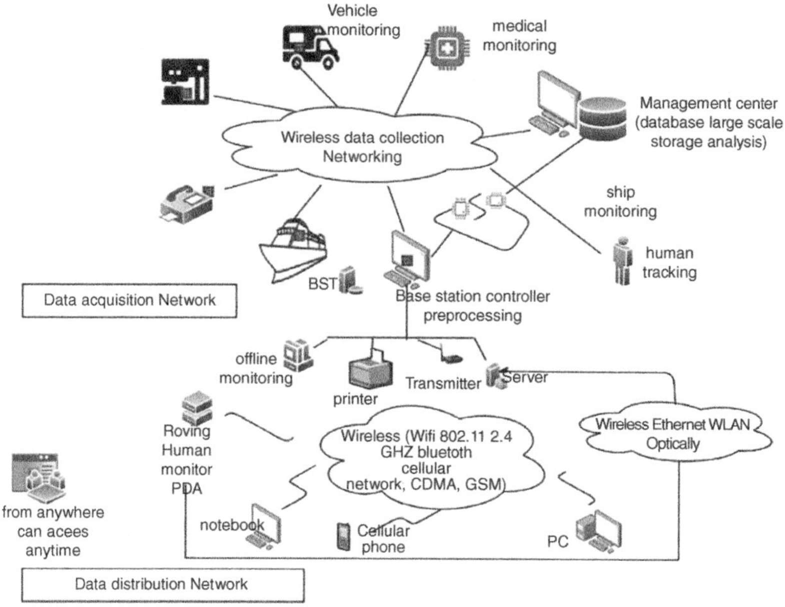

Figure 7.2 Wireless sensor network.

are used to measure conditions or variables such as sound or pressure and send the corresponding data to the base station, as shown in Figure 7.2.

7.1.2.1 Types of Different WSNs

Based on the surroundings, the different types of WSN networks needed are determined on the basis of where they are employed such as land, underwater, or underground. The various types of WSNs include [8]:

7.1.2.1.1 Terrestrial WSNs This type of WSNs has the ability to communicate mean exchange or share with gateway productively. It essentially includes pre-planned (structured) or ad hoc (unstructured) ways 100 to 1000 wireless sensor nodes. In a pre-planned manner consider are organized in 2D, 3D, grid, and optimal placement patterns, and in Ad hoc, i.e. In an unstructured manner, the sensor is arranged randomly towards the target area, further in a fixed plane.

In this type of WSN, the battery capacity is very small or limited, and the batteries receive secondary power from solar cells. The consumption of low

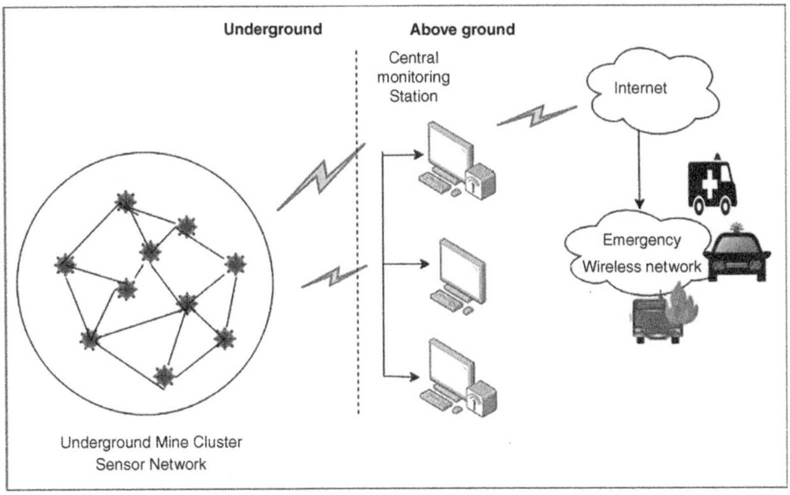

Figure 7.3 Underground WSNs.

energy of these types of WSNs can be achieved further using reduce delays, optimal routing, low duty cycle, and so on [9].

7.1.2.1.2 Underground WSNs To detect underground movement or conditions, several types of sensor nodes are hidden under the ground in this type of WSNs system. Further, to transfer the data to the base station via sensor nodes, additional nodes are added as sink nodes above the surface of the ground, as shown in Figure 7.3. The terrestrial types of WSN are cheaper than the alternative underground WSNs, as in underground WSNs deployment and maintenance are costly.

In this, the batteries are difficult to recharge as they are underground; this is especially problematic for the sensors, which have limited battery power. It is a big challenge to maintain the network as there is a substantial signal loss and attenuation problems [8].

7.1.2.1.3 Underwater WSNs As we all know, 70% of our earth is covered with water. In underwater WSNs, the sensor nodes and vehicles are employed underwater, to keep an eye on the underwater conditions, as shown in Figure 7.4. Autonomous vehicles help in gathering data or information from the sensor link nodes and sending it to the base station. Underwater communication is very challenging, which leads to risks such as bandwidth and long propagation delay and sometimes sensor failures too.

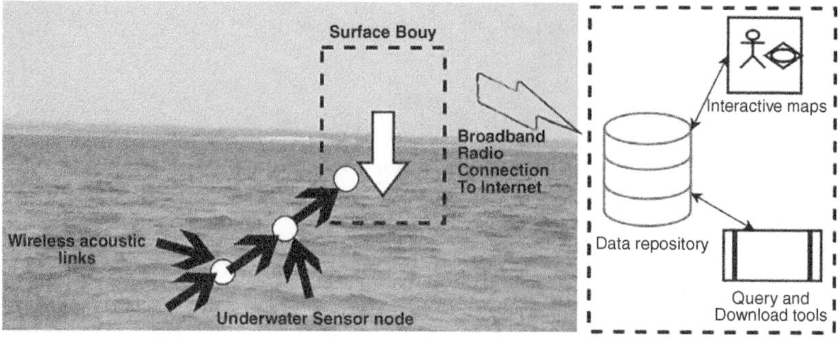

Figure 7.4 Underwater WSNs.

In these networks, a big disadvantage is that we cannot replace or recharge batteries easily. Further energy conservation issues in underwater WSNs involve the developments in networking techniques and underwater communication techniques.

7.1.2.1.4 Multimedia WSNs In this type of WSNs, the monitoring and tracking of events are done in the form of multimedia, such as audio, imaging, and video, as shown in Figure 7.5. In these networks low-rate cost sensors are employed, which are equipped with cameras and microphones; this makes these networks cheap. Through a wireless connection, nodes can communicate with each other for data compression, retrieval, and correlation. The challenge with these networks is that their energy consumption is very high, due to their high bandwidth, data processing,

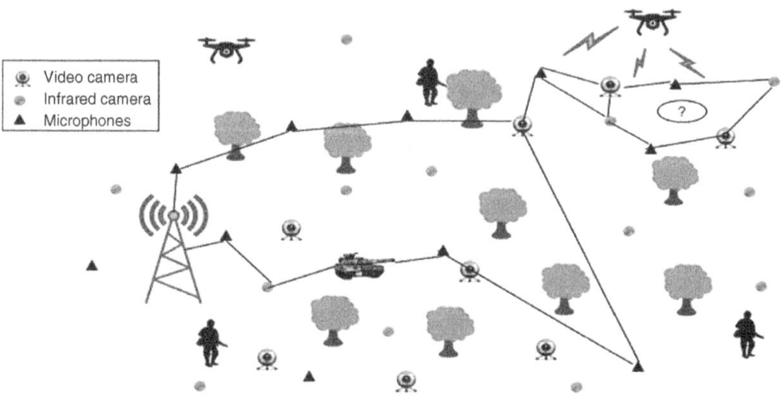

Figure 7.5 Multimedia WSNs.

and compressing techniques. High bandwidth is used to deliver content easily and efficiently [9].

7.1.2.1.5 Mobile WSNs As the word "mobile" means moveable, in mobile WSNs (MWSNs) the sensors can move autonomously to interact with the different physical environments. Further, these networks have the capability to communicate and compute independently.

As compared to a fixed wireless network, mobile wireless networks are more versatile. The advantage of MWSNs as compared to static or fixed networks is that their coverage is better, they have superior channel capacity, and they have better energy efficiency, among others [7].

7.1.2.2 Constraints of Wireless Sensor Networks

- Very limited storage capacity (up to 100 KB)
- Modest processing power (up to 8 MHz)
- Consumes more power in communication over a short range
- Requires minimum energy with constrain in the protocol
- Short battery life
- Inactive devices deliver minute energy

7.1.2.3 Applications of Wireless Sensor Networks

Applications of WSNs include the following, which are shown in Figure 7.6.

- WSNs are used for environment monitoring and tracking, such as tracking of animals, forest detection, weather forecasting, and flood detection.

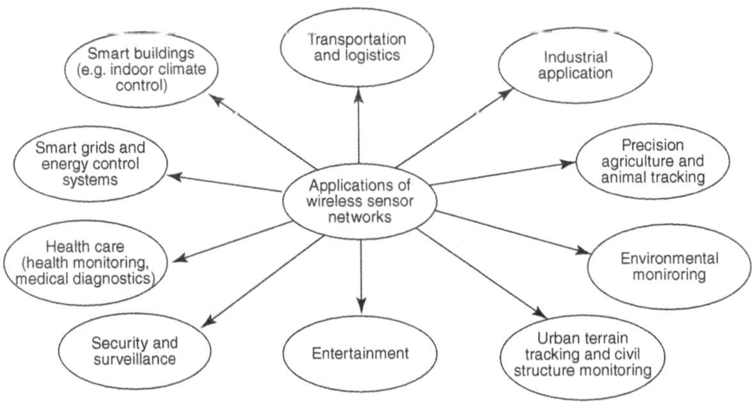

Figure 7.6 Applications of wireless sensor networks.

Further, they are also used as commercial applications for prediction, monitoring, and detection of seismic activities [10].

- Military-based application of WSNs include environment monitoring, temperature, humidity, and tracking of objects, which act as a surveillance system. The user can remotely control the sensor links using a sensor-based network, which is dropped to a field of investigation; from this network, the enemy can be easily tracked, and any movement of the object can be detected [11].
- Health-based applications of these networks are tracking and monitoring of patients; these networks are used by doctors [10–12].
- The most recurrent use of WSN-based applications is in the field of transport or vehicle systems, which include parking monitoring, traffic monitoring, and dynamic routing management. [10].
- The other varieties of this network include industrial process monitoring, rapid emergency response, ecosystem and habitat monitoring, automated building climate control, civil infrastructure structural health monitoring. [11–12].

7.1.3 WSNs as a Subset of IoT

IoT is at a higher stage of development than WSNs; sometimes, WSN technology can also be used within an IoT system. As in a mesh network, a large number of sensors are employed to gather data individually and transfer this data to the Internet via the router in an IoT system.

The work should not consider the "wireless sensor or Wi-Fi" as the "Internet of things." Wireless networks include only the wireless sensor, but any network that includes the wired sensor is no longer known as a wireless sensor or Wi-Fi network. It is unlike IoT. Any object or device connected to or related to the Internet is considered an IoT device. An IoT system is thus elucidated as a group of multiple IoT devices [13].

Examples

- A fridge having the capacity of sending temperature readings to the Internet should not be considered as a WSN, but it is an IoT device.
- A large collection of sensors used to monitor rain on an acre of land is likely to be considered a WSN, as all the sensors are wireless. This system may or may not be connected to an IoT system.

Today's applications based on network computing are faced with a huge demand for powerful functionalities networks. The reach of the functional network is central to customer satisfaction both in cloud computing and mobile network environments. WSN is a wireless or Wi-Fi network containing objects or stand-alone spatial diffusion devices using sensors for careful physical monitoring or environmental conditions, such as sound, humidity, temperature, pressure, vibration, motion or pollutants, at various different area or locations.

A WSN is a collection of sensing devices that can communicate wirelessly. By this generation of technology, sensing elements have become the most important object. Sensors are small and perfect for the features of sensing motion, pressure, and human touch and even the atmospheric temperature. The small size and light weight are the best advantages of sensors that help to design a device. The fetched data of sensors are processed with the help of open-source license platform Arduino IDE (integrated development environment). Arduino IDE is open-source license computer software. ThingSpeak is a cloud-based platform used to store the sensor data in the cloud and is also an open-source license platform.

7.1.4 Motivation and Organization of the Chapter

Our motivation is the lack of sufficient research in the area of smart surveillance systems for patients with closed-loop alarm in the field of WSNs. This motivation helps us to implement experimentation based on IoT- and WSNs-based smart surveillance systems for patients with closed-loop alarm.

Implementing real-time data recovery from various wireless sensors and storing this data on a cloud-based platform called ThingSpeak. Various sensors are used to measure pulse, acceleration, SpO2 (oxygen saturation), and temperature for this experiment. The purpose of using the pulse sensor is to detect the heart rate. Acceleration sensors are used to detect movement or acceleration of the individual. SpO2 sensors are used to measure the amount of oxygen present in the blood, or simply the percentage of hemoglobin containing oxygen. The temperature sensor is used to detect the body temperature. Before sending any data to the cloud, first the data need to be fetched from the sensors in real time. In our experiment, the output of fetched data in real time were stored in the cloud and shown in the Android application in a closed loop. The experimental results are explained briefly in the next section.

This chapter is divided into five sections. Section 7.1 illustrates the introduction of the IoT and WSNs with its applications and working principles. Section 7.2 constitutes the literature review related to different phases and techniques of health-monitoring systems (HMSs) and their relation to IoT and WSNs for choosing the correct vital sign sensors for patients' HMSs. Section 7.3 describes the proposed research of WSNs and IoT-based smart surveillance systems for patients with closed-loop alarms; it also describes the research methodology. Section 7.4 provides an evaluation of the proposed methodology; it discusses the entire experimental environments. Further, the results and outcomes of patient-monitoring smart surveillance systems are clearly shown graphically and diagrammatically. Section 7.5 includes the conclusion and future scope in the results in terms of a patient-monitoring smart surveillance system based on WSNs and IoT devices.

7.2 Literature Review

The literature studied for this chapter mainly focused on the application of IoT and WSNs based on patient-monitoring systems; the literature concludes that these technologies improve real-time monitoring systems for the patient in removed locations. In the literature review, the authors have discussed all the modern as well as old techniques applied in the field of IoT and WSNs for monitoring from 2012 to 2020.

7.2.1 Literature Review: Toward the Application of IoT and WSNs

Mitra et al. [14] discuss a system that is based on the KNOWME platform for real-time health monitoring. KNOWME is further integrated with the N95 Nokia phone. The main purpose of the paper was to evaluate and monitor four major challenges. These four challenges are as follows: (i) achieving strength in the subject-induced changeability in terms of sensor placement or mobility for the environment operates, (ii) minimizing the consumption of network energy and balancing the strain while acquiring top fidelity information, (iii) using modest sensors enabling precise physical movement detection, and (iv) at last designing WBANs to resolve the physiological quantity of the concentration similar to energy expenditures.

Patel et al. [15] review the technology based on wireless systems and sensors in the field of treatment. The study is focused on wearable sensors systems and their various applications such as disorders detection at an early age, safety, wellness and health, assessment of treatment efficacy, and home treatment. The authors have also described the monitoring of adults of older age groups with unrelieved conditions in terms of ambient and wearable sensors.

Kothari et al. [16] review the developments in the field of WSNs, its applications, and design constraints, which also include a lifetime evaluation model. The model is based on a multi-parameter monitoring system in real time, with the help of LabView graphical programming language and a microcontroller such as ZigBee. Distance and temperature are the two-parameter analog information gained by the system; with the help of ZigBee the information is transmitted to the other end, i.e., the receiver side.

Hackmann et al. [17] discuss the deterioration of civil infrastructure, the need for structural health monitoring, and the critical challenge of localization and detection of damage. Further, the discussion results in two conclusions: (i) there is a trade-off between resolution and various sensors in terms of localization damage process based on elasticity, and (ii) based on energy efficiency based on elasticity, multi-level planned calculation structural design. The authors also perform a simulation to explain the complete structure that displays the effectiveness of the system in damage localization and energy-effectiveness as well as truss structure.

Misra et al. [18] present a theoretical model of the cloud-sensor platform and a mathematical formulation cloud-based sensor according to their virtualization characteristics. The researchers mainly focus on the challenges and ideology of WSN applications and their behavior in terms of a cloud-sensor platform. At last, in the results, the authors confirm the lifecycle of the sensors, which increase by 3.25%, energy consumption decreases by 36.68%.

Simoes and de Souza [19] discuss a communication technique known as data acquisition system (DAS) in place of north 52° SOS execution of OGC SWE specification. Further, this enables interoperability and interaction of web sensors. At last, the authors come with the result of a low-cost programmed DAS system for town sites humidity and a temperature-monitoring system build in IoT. For the future, the authors also provide a complete infrastructure for visualizing information in the concrete background of Big Data and derived from IoT.

Zakaria and Michael [20] present a prototype to monitor pH, the dissolved parameter of oxygen, and conductivity from water waste, which is discharged into water sources, with the help of a cloud-based integrated WSNs environment. It uses the capability of IoT, which provides the system the ability to online monitor it in real time and upload the sensor data or information in the cloud-based platform, named ThingSpeak. The authors use the GPRS service to transfer the data into the cloud with the help of AT commands in combination with the HTTP GET protocol. The prototype used a Telerivet SMS gateway to report experiential or acknowledged water pollution using alert notification by SMS.

Xie et al. [21] propose a routing implementation of efficient energy that introduces mobility of the objects with WSNs for collection information of mobile data. The term used for sensing moveable sensors is mobile data collectors (MDCs). MDCs start the movement of data from its initial place-based station and transfer the data periodically to all the stations and finally return to the base station again. This whole movement of data from one station to another is decided using the Floyd-Warshall complete graph algorithm.

Chandra et al. [22] discuss data-driven techniques that help improve yields in agriculture. Moreover, this technology has a high rate of manual information gathering in bare implementation and gives a limited connectivity result. The authors present an uninterrupted IoT platform known as FarmBeats for agriculture solutions to collect data from various drones, cameras, and sensors. FareBeats is a method that helps in monitoring cabs through the Internet and has been implemented six months ago in two US farms.

Miqdad et al. [23] developed a real-time low-cost WSNs monitoring system for sensing building space. The monitoring system collects data such as temperature, illumination, quality of air, and humidity. The collection of data is taken from all corners of the building to balance the amount of energy and client comfort to accomplish the goal. In the experiment, the authors use the NodeMCU module with a DHT11 sensor for measuring humidity and temperature. 6 V power supply sources are used to supply power to the NodeMCU module.

AlSkaif et al. [24] compare environment monitoring of smart cities in four specific areas: smart building/house, smart animal and agriculture farming, and municipal resilience. The main aim of the research is to carry out a comparative analysis of the MAC protocol, the use of energy in low-throughput MSN data networks (wireless multimedia sensor networks). In comparison, the analysis includes the multi-class traffic model for analyzing the energy usage of the MAC protocol in low-speed data.

Modieginyane et al. [25] review the challenges faced in applications for environmental monitoring by WSNs in addition to challenges faced by opportunities and approaches. The study elaborates on how an application released helps to resolve the opportunities and approaches related to WSNs with the help of SDN.

Sethi and Sahoo [26] propose an application based on a health-monitoring system (HMS). The application is purely based on WSNs, which help to monitor the medical information or record in real time. The role of the application is to collect data from adult patients, ICU, and industrial uses. In the experiment the authors use ZigBee and Wi-Fi to transfer the data to the application.

Kaur et al. [27] discuss the effective role of IoT in the field of healthcare devices. The IoT-based devices provide patient health state and track their activities according to the current time and situation. Further, given a viewpoint in the field of electronics and technology, which is fussing together into the Internet of healthcare Things (IoHT). Finally, the authors aim to provide benefits of IoHT in the medical sector.

7.3 Proposed Work: WSN and IoT-Based Smart Surveillance System for Patients with Closed-Loop Alarm

Numerous studies have been conducted on HMS but not much has been published on closed-loop real-time patients' HMS. This study will propose and focus on an enhanced monitoring system for patients based on IoT and WSNs with closed-loop alarm. This implementation of a closed-loop patient-monitoring system was done using four vital sign sensors (SpO2 sensor, accelerometer, thermometer, and pulse sensor), as shown in Figure 7.7. The closed-loop patient-monitoring system consists of three different phases. The first phase is to connect the entire vital sensor together in a device to measure different parameters. The temperature sensor is used to measure the body temperature in degrees Celsius as well as Fahrenheit. SpO2 (oxygen saturation) is used to measure the amount of oxygen present in hemoglobin in the blood of the person's body in percentage units. The accelerometer sensor is used to measure the acceleration of the body and to determine the state that the body is in. At last, a pulse

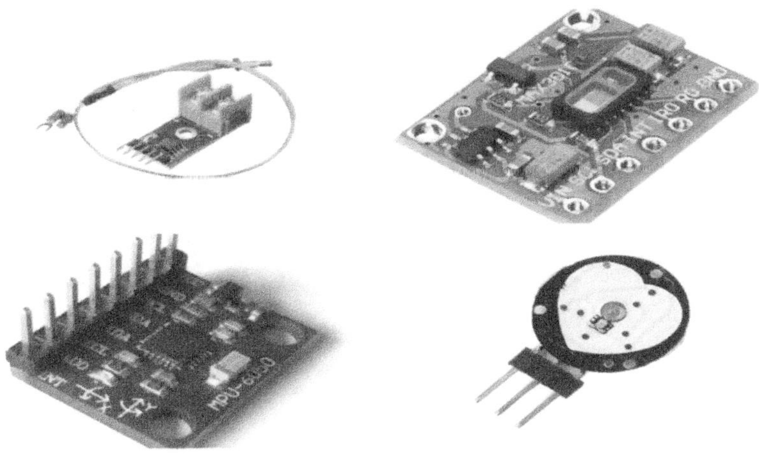

Figure 7.7 Sensors used in experiments.

sensor is used in the experiment to measure the heart rate of the person in beats per minute (BPM).

The second phase is to send the sensors data into the cloud platform. The cloud platform used in the experiment is ThingSpeak. The reason for choosing the ThingSpeak web-based cloud is that it is open source for used till four channels and is provided by MathWorks, the company that makes MATLAB. In ThingSpeak, data can easily be transferred using an application programming interface (API) key and channels ID. Finally, the final phase of the experiment is to create an Android-based application, which uses the ParseInt method to collect the sensors data from the cloud into an Android application in real time. Figure 7.8 shows the proposed architecture model.

7.3.1 Methodology

There are basically four phases that will be used to complete the research objectives.

The first phase is identifying all wireless sensors used in vital signs according to their efficiency of giving constant results, cost, reliability, and power consumption. Choosing each sensor was done using various experiments. After the selection process, the data of the sensors first view in the serial monitor of the Arduino IDE. Then the data are sent to the ThingSpeak cloud platform.

The second phase is to interface all the sensors together in a compact device. This device basically consists of one D1 WeMos mini microcontroller, also known as Mini NodeMCU, along with four vital sign sensors.

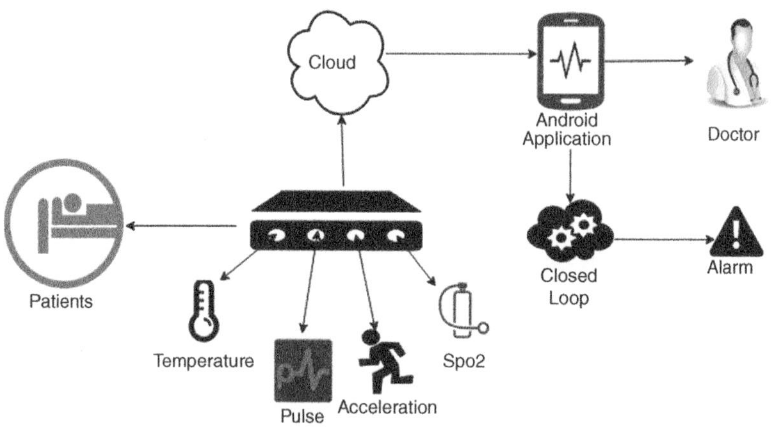

Figure 7.8 The proposed model architecture.

The third phase is to fetch all the sensor data from the ThingSpeak cloud platform to an Android application in a closed loop. The closed-loop alarm is a process in which two thresholds are set (upper and lower), and if the actual value is in between them, that means it's in normal condition; otherwise it will activate an alert. The application used the parseInt method to fetch the JSON format data from the cloud.

The fourth and final phase is to implement and test the device in real time by attaching the four sensors together in the body of a person, to check the accuracy, efficiency, and reliability of the device in different conditions.

Altogether the above phases are now shown and explained in Figure 7.9 using a flowchart.

The steps of Figure 7.9 start with the related survey in the field of WSNs and IoT. In the survey, the authors explore existing WSNs and IoT-based VST (vital sign transmission) concerning cloud having a closed-loop application. In the conclusion, the authors identified the four sensors needed in VST for patient-monitoring systems; these are an SpO2 sensor, accelerometer, temperature sensor, and pulse sensor. The sensors are attached to a device in a compact form; all the sensors are connected to a D1-mini NodeMCU microcontroller. The controller has an built-in Wi-Fi module; the module helps to transfer the data of the sensor to the cloud using the Arduino IDE. The ThingSpeak a web-based cloud platform is used to store the data of the sensors. The data is further sent to an Android-based application using the parseInt method; the application also consists of a closed-loop alert system. Closed loop is set based on the thresholds for both upper and lower bounds so that if the value is below or above the min or max thresholds, respectively, it will give an alert. Different threshold values are set according to the sensor so that each sensor has its own thresholds. The alert can be viewed as color-changing effects in a text box, where sensor data, if seen in the application, is displayed in the results and discussion section of the following chapter. The data is on JSON format when it is stored in the ThingSpeak cloud platform. Using the API key and channel ID of the ThingSpeak server of an individual, the data is shared in a link, as shown in Figures 7.10–7.12. Further, the link is used in the Android application to fetch the data from the cloud.

The ParseInt method is used to extract the value of each JSON format data of each sensor. This data can be viewed anywhere using the application; it will help the doctor to view the details of the patients in real time from anywhere. The doctor can take necessary action before the patient reaches the medical.

The testing of the devices is done based on their compatibility, usability, security, reliability and scalability, performance, and data integrity. Let's explore each testing type one by one.

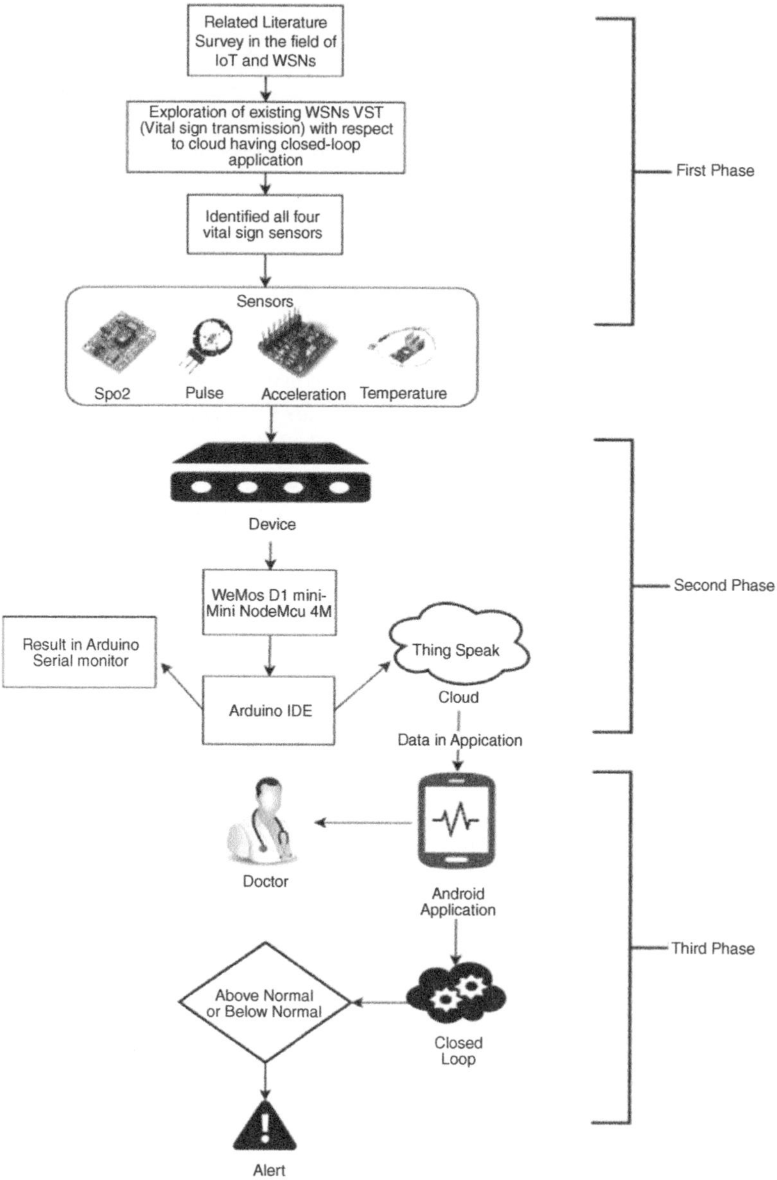

Figure 7.9 Methodology flowchart.

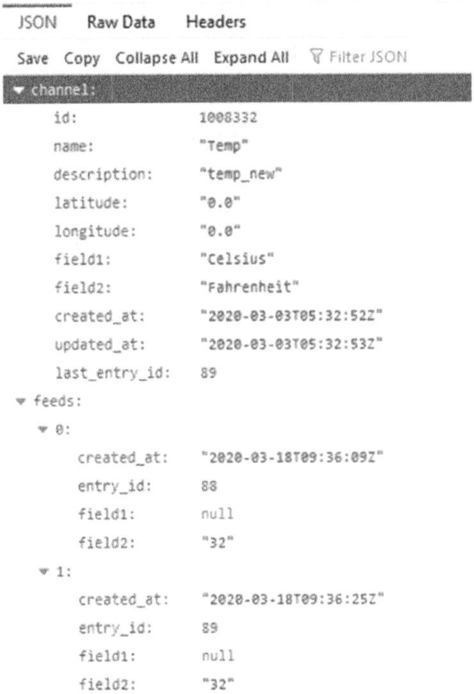

Figure 7.10 Channel details.

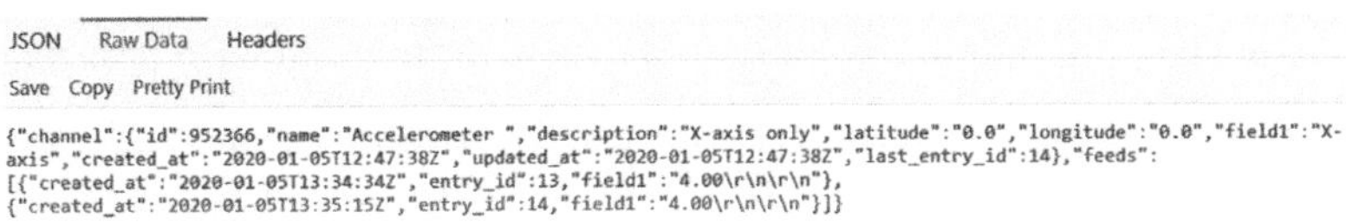

Figure 7.11 Raw data.

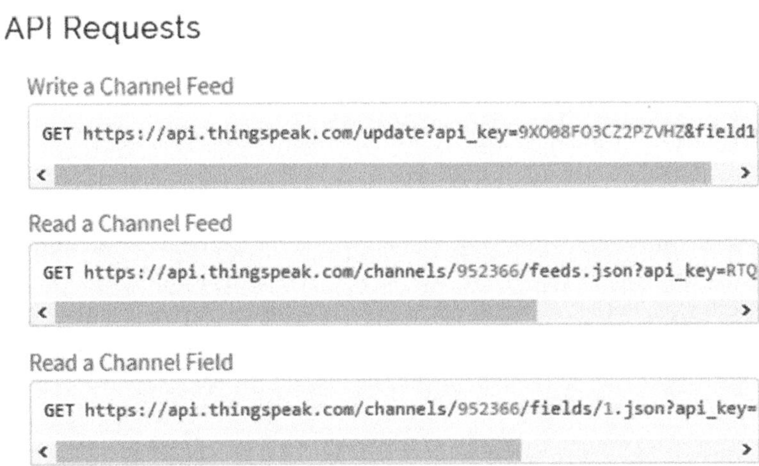
API Requests
Write a Channel Feed
GET https://api.thingspeak.com/update?api_key=9XO08FO3CZ2PZVHZ&field1
Read a Channel Feed
GET https://api.thingspeak.com/channels/952366/feeds.json?api_key=RTQ
Read a Channel Field
GET https://api.thingspeak.com/channels/952366/fields/1.json?api_key=

Figure 7.12 Link to read a channel feed [28].

- **Usability of the Device**
  The user interface of the application is checked, considering one too many users, according to their comfort to read the data and the ease to access the application.
- **Compatibility Testing**
  As the system is composed of hardware as well as software, the configuration of both together is tested so that it can give an accurate result. Compatibility is one of the most important parts of an IoT-based device.
- **Scalability and Reliability Testing**
  Scalability and reliability of the sensor are tested continuously running the devices for a long time. Basically, in this test the breaking point of the sensor is found out so that when it runs in real time it won't face any problem.
- **The Integrity of Data Testing**
  In IoT device testing, it is very important to test the integrity of the data, as a large amount of data is involved in the application, continuously checking whether the data measured by the sensor is the same or not.
- **Security Testing of the Device**
  Security in terms of accessing the application of the device, security should be provided so that only the authenticated user can see the data or access the application. Providing validation to the user can solve this kind of issue.
- **Performance Testing**
  Testing should be performed in each step of the IoT-based device to make sure that it is running correctly and giving accurate result in each phase.

7.4 Implementation and Evaluation of the WSN and IoT-Based Smart Surveillance System for Patients with Closed-Loop Alarm

7.4.1 Experimental Environment

An experimental environment plays a very important part in performing the experiment. Each experiment depends entirely on the subject of the experiment, since it is the primary source of all the results. This experience involves a number of components such as sensors, Wi-Fi modules, Arduino IDE; cloud-based open-source platform. A brief description of all requirements can be found below.

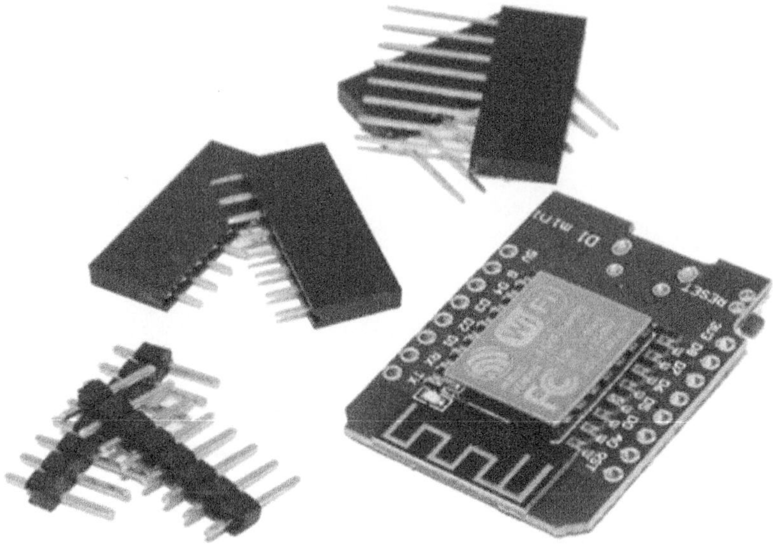

Figure 7.13 WeMos D1 mini – Mini NodeMcu [29].

7.4.1.1 Wi-Fi Module

Among many Wi-Fi modules, WeMos D1 mini – Mini NodeMCU is used for this experiment. As shown in Figure 7.13, D1 mini NodeMCU is small and functional, but here the purpose of using this module is sending sensor data to the cloud. One of the great features of the Wi-Fi module is its wireless Internet connection. D1 mini NodeMCU is an IoT-based ready-made open-source platform. The power supply required to run this controller is 5V or 3.3V.

7.4.1.2 Sensors

This experiment includes various sensors to measure variables such as SpO2, pulse, temperature, and acceleration.

The temperature sensor model number MAX6675 is used to measure the body temperature in degrees Celsius and as well as Fahrenheit. SpO2 (oxygen saturation) module number MAX30102 is used to measure the amount of oxygen present in hemoglobin in the blood, as previously explained. An accelerometer is used to detect the acceleration in all three axes, i.e., the x-, y-, and z-axis. At last, a pulse sensor is used in the experiment to measure the heart rate of the person.

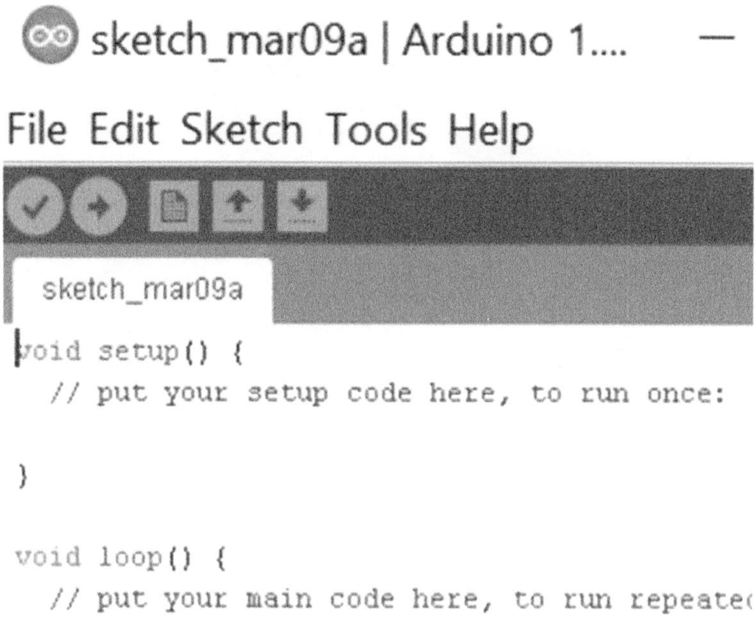

Figure 7.14 Ardunio IDE software [30].

7.4.1.3 Arduino IDE

This software is open-source, user-friendly, and free. All real-time data of various sensors are fetched in Arduino IDE using computer programming, as shown in Figure 7.14

7.4.1.4 ThingSpeak

This is a cloud-based, open-source platform. It is shown in Figure 7.15. In this platform, real-time data of any objects can be sent and stored as a representation of a graph. Sending and storing data on this platform requires

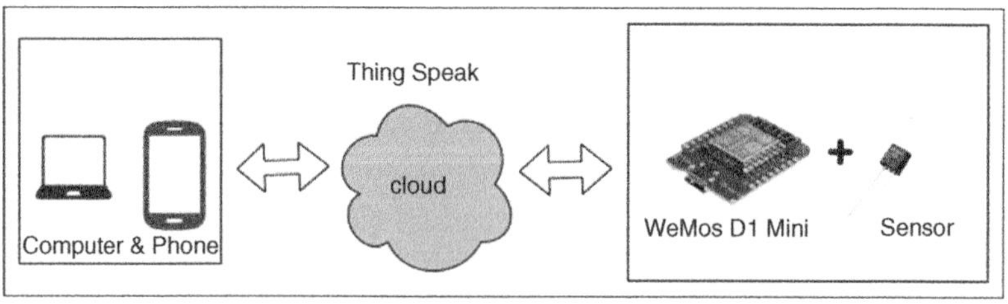

Figure 7.15 ThingSpeak IoT platform [31].

any Wi-Fi or Bluetooth modules. According to the requirement, D1 mini WeMos NodeMCU was chosen as a Wi-Fi module to implement this experiment.

7.4.2 Results and Discussion

This implementation was done using four sensors (SpO2, acceleration, temperature, and pulse) in two different steps. The first step was to perform individual connectivity of all sensors one by one with their individual outputs. The second step was to make one connection with all four sensors to get one output with different sensors in the cloud. The real-time data was fetched by WeMos D1 mini and stored in ThingSpeak. The authors studied all the resources and technology before starting the implementation. Figure 7.16 shows the architecture of all the components and how the connection is made. All the steps of this experiment are explained with their results.

7.4.2.1 SpO2

The experiment began with SpO2 and followed by the three other variables, i.e., pulse, temperature, and acceleration. The use of SpO2 is to measure the amount of oxygen present in the blood, or simply the percentage of hemoglobin contains oxygen.

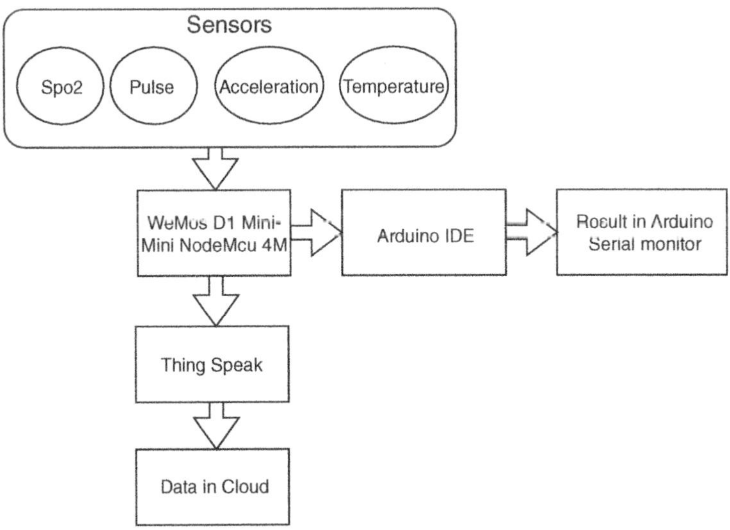

Figure 7.16 Connection architecture of all the components.

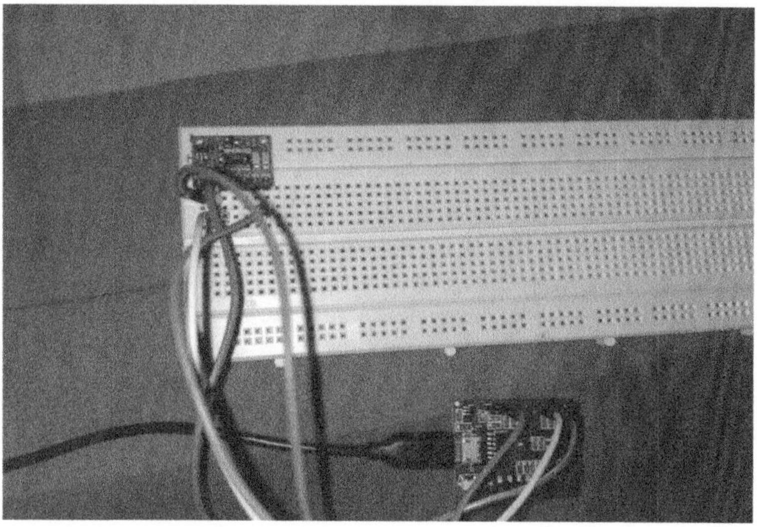

Figure 7.17 MAX30102 pulse oximeter/heart-rate sensor.

The SpO2 data is fetched in real time, and then the output is shown in the Arduino IDE. Figures 7.17 and 7.18 show the connection of the SpO2 sensor with the WeMos D1 mini-module and the output in the Arduino IDE, respectively.

7.4.2.2 Pulse

A heart-rate sensor, or pulse sensor, is used to sense the BPM of the person. The real-time BPM data was fetched by connecting the pulse sensor with the WeMos D1 mini-module. Figures 7.19 and 7.20 show how the pulse sensor was connected with the Wi-Fi module and the fetched data as output in the Arduino IDE, respectively.

7.4.2.3 Acceleration

To get acceleration data, the authors used an accelerometer. This sensor can fetch the acceleration data in all three axes, i.e., the x-, y-, and z-axis. Figures 7.21 and 7.22 show the connection of the accelerometer with the Wi-Fi module and the output in the Arduino IDE, respectively.

7.4.2.4 Temperature

The authors used the MAX6675 temperature sensor. MAX6675 was found suitable for implementing this experiment to sensing the temperature because it is small in size and gives accurate results. The real-time

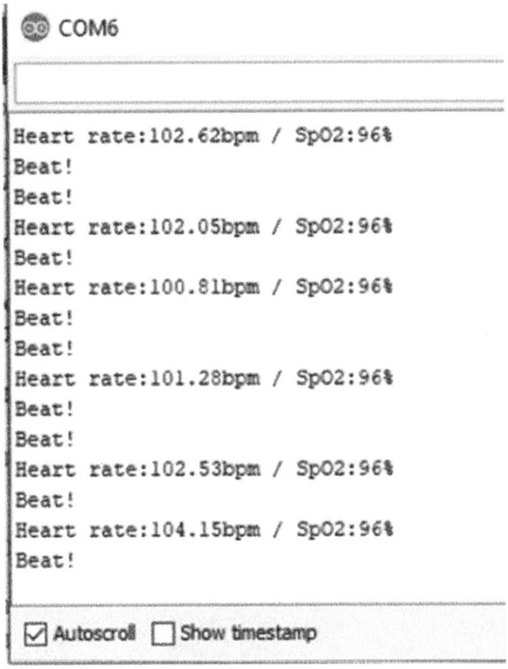

Figure 7.18 MAX30102 pulse oximeter sensor data in Arduino IDE.

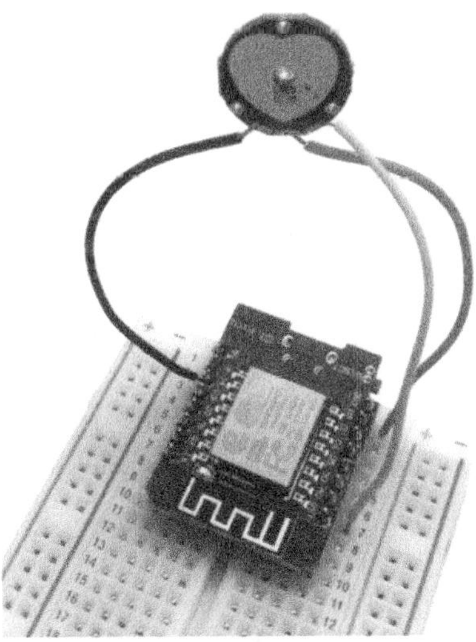

Figure 7.19 Pulse sensor.

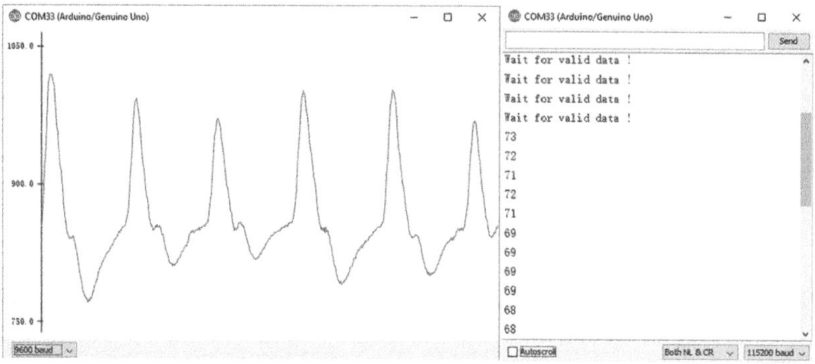

Figure 7.20 Pulse sensor data in Arduino IDE.

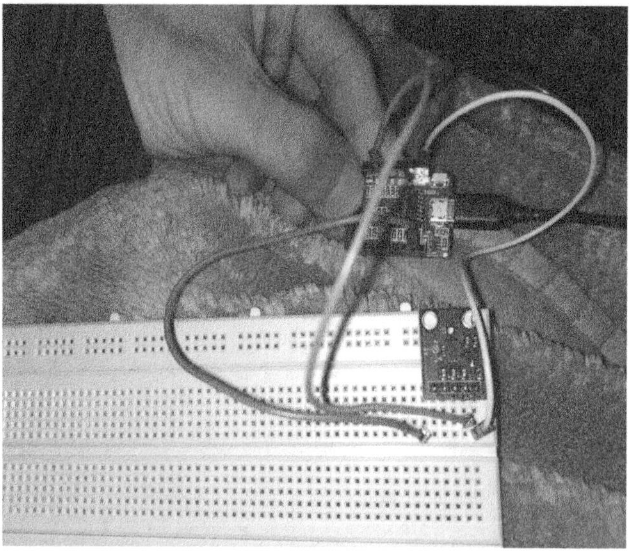

Figure 7.21 Accelerometer sensor.

temperature data was fetched by connecting the MAX6675 sensor with the WeMos D1 mini-module. Figures 7.23 and 7.24 show how MAX6675 was connected with the Wi-Fi module and the fetched data as output in the Arduino IDE, respectively.

7.4.2.5 Combined

After completing the first step, this part includes the process of fetching all four sensors' data in one connection with the WeMos D1 mini-module and showing their outputs in ThingSpeak. However, after getting the data from

```
x-axis= 303        y-axis= 304        z-axis= 302
x-axis= 303        y-axis= 304        z-axis= 302
x-axis= 303        y-axis= 303        z-axis= 301
x-axis= 303        y-axis= 303        z-axis= 301
x-axis= 303        y-axis= 304        z-axis= 302
x-axis= 304        y-axis= 304        z-axis= 302
x-axis= 303        y-axis= 304        z-axis= 302
x-axis= 303        y-axis= 304        z-axis= 302
x-axis= 302        y-axis= 302        z-axis= 300
x-axis= 300        y-axis= 300        z-axis= 299
x-axis= 299        y-axis= 299        z-axis= 298
x-axis= 299        y-axis= 300        z-axis= 298
x-axis= 300        y-axis= 300        z-axis= 298
x-axis= 300        y-axis= 300        z-axis= 298
x-axis= 300        y-axis= 300        z-axis= 298
x-axis= 300        y-axis= 300        z-axis= 298
```

☐ Autoscroll

Figure 7.22 Accelerometer data in Arduino IDE.

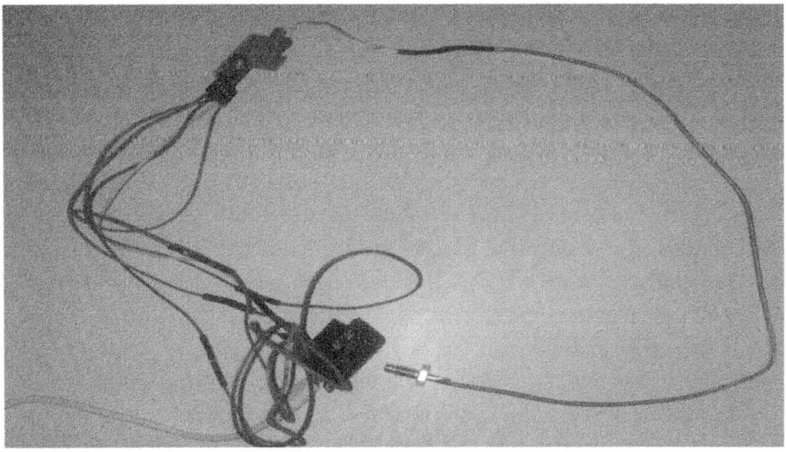

Figure 7.23 MAX6675 sensor data in Arduino IDE.

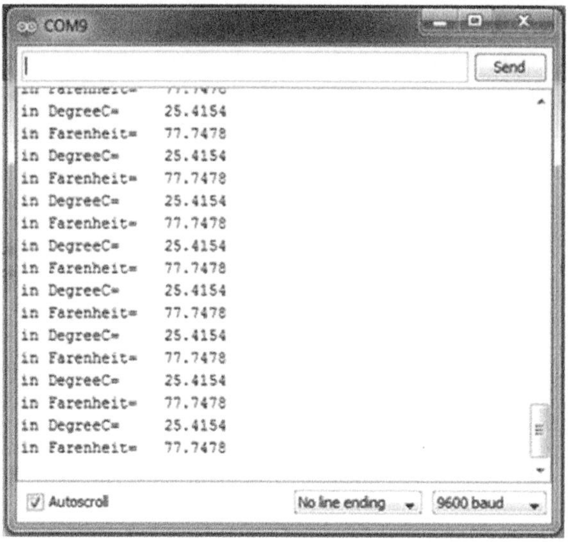

Figure 7.24 MAX6675 sensor data in Arduino IDE.

all four sensors, the main process is to send the data to the cloud. The WeMos D1 mini Wi-Fi module was found suitable for this experiment because it is easy to work with. Figures 7.17–7.24 show the connection of all four sensors with the WeMos D1 mini-module. Figures 7.24 and 7.25 show the result of the MAX30102 pulse oximeter sensor, which, as previously explained, was sent to the cloud using ThingSpeak represented as a graph. Figure 7.26 shows the output of the MAX6675 temperature sensor in the graph form. Figure 7.27 shows the output of the accelerometer, where (a), (b), and (c) represent the acceleration in the x-, y-, and z-axis, respectively. At last, Figure 7.28 shows the result of pulse sensor data sent to the cloud using ThingSpeak in the form of a graph.

ThingSpeak stores data represented as a graph. The user needs to create an account in ThingSpeak, and then ThingSpeak will provide the cloud services. Figures 7.28 are the final results of this execution, which were sent to the cloud. In the Arduino IDE different programming codes were used to get the results from each sensor by connecting with the WeMos D1 mini-module. A wireless network mobile hotspot was used for Internet connection in this experiment.

Finally, at the last steps of the implementation, data was sent from the cloud to an Android application. Android applications are a very popular source of IoT software, which loads up mobile devices to operate and act as a middleware for interaction between users and the devices. In this

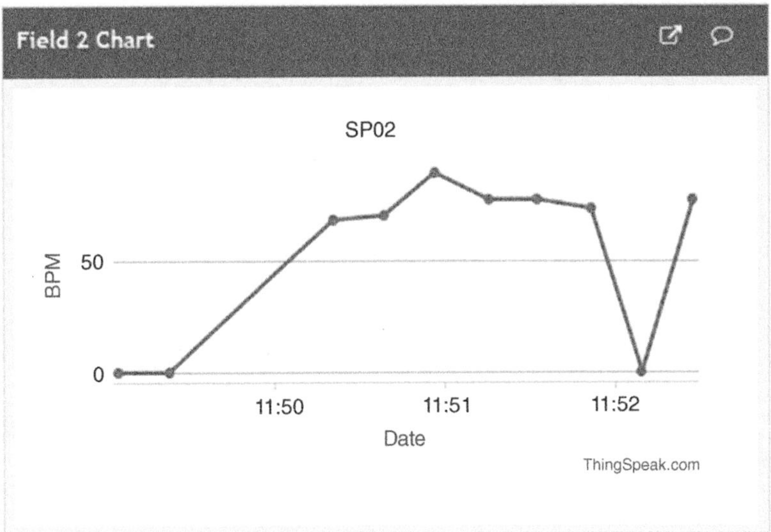

Figure 7.25 MAX30102 pulse oximeter sensor data in ThingSpeak.

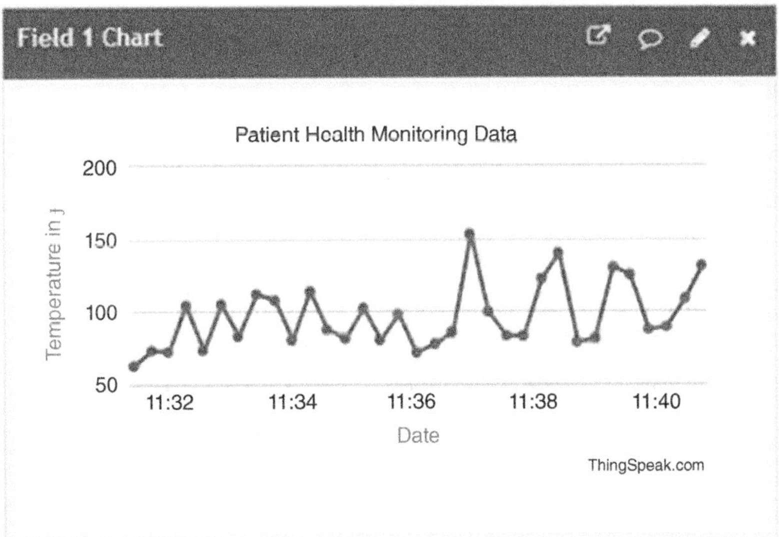

Figure 7.26 Temperature sensor data in ThingSpeak.

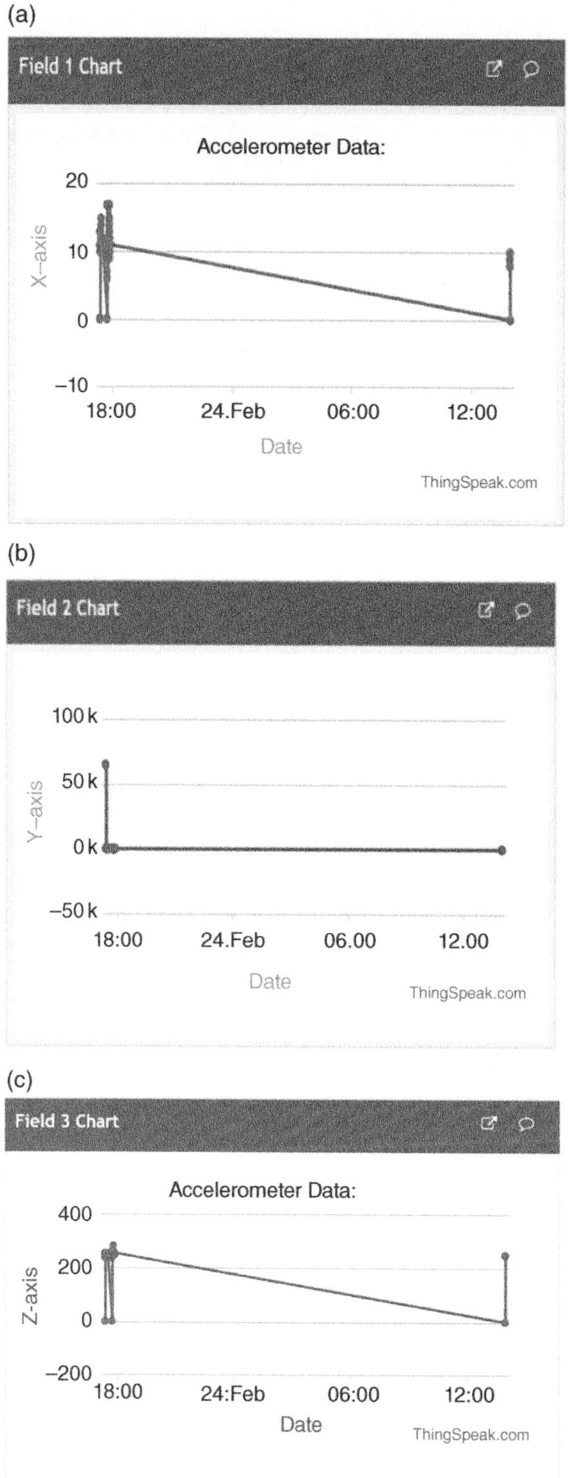

Figure 7.27 (a) Data of accelerometer of x-axis sent in ThingSpeak. (b) Data of accelerometer of y-axis sent in ThingSpeak. (c) Data of accelerometer of z-axis sent in ThingSpeak

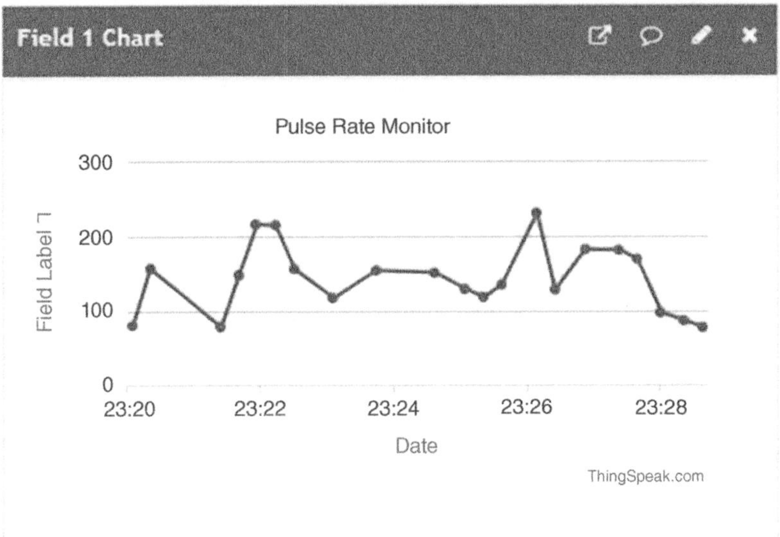

Figure 7.28 Pulse sensor data in ThingSpeak.

experiment the Android application acts as middleware between a doctor who used the application for reading the patient's data in real time from anywhere. Reading of the data from the cloud to the Android application is done using the parseInt method. In this method a JSON link is used to fetch the different data, further, this data is displayed in a textbox in the application. The application also has a closed-loop alert system, which helps to notify the user of any major change in the reading of the data. For operating the application, the user needs to sign in, or if the user is not registered yet, they need to sing up as a new user, as shown in Figure 7.29.

After successfully logging in, the user will navigate to the patient's data interface, where all sensors' data is shown in each textbox, such as pulse, acceleration, SpO2, and temperature in degrees Celsius. Figure 7.30 shows the reading of a patient's data in an Android application from the cloud.

The alert notification is visible in the patient's data interface with the help of color-changing effects in the textbox for each particular text field, when the value of the variable is outside a predetermined range, as previously explained. Figure 7.31 shows the patient's data with the alert notification.

This whole technology can be used for any emergency, such as patients who are in transit mode, in ambulances. The doctor can easily start to

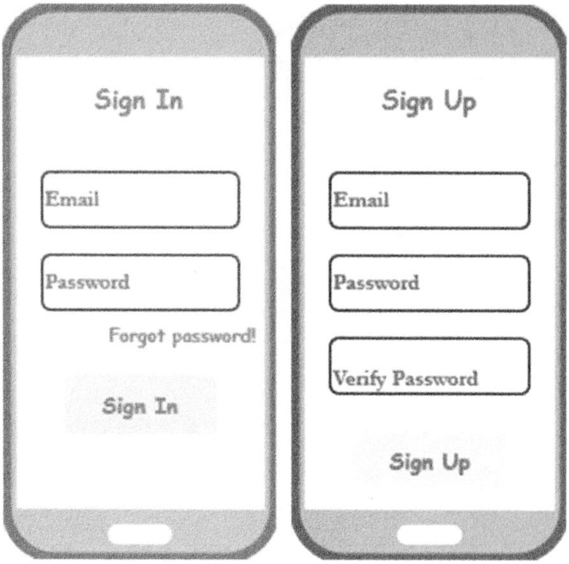

Figure 7.29 Sign-In/-Up interface.

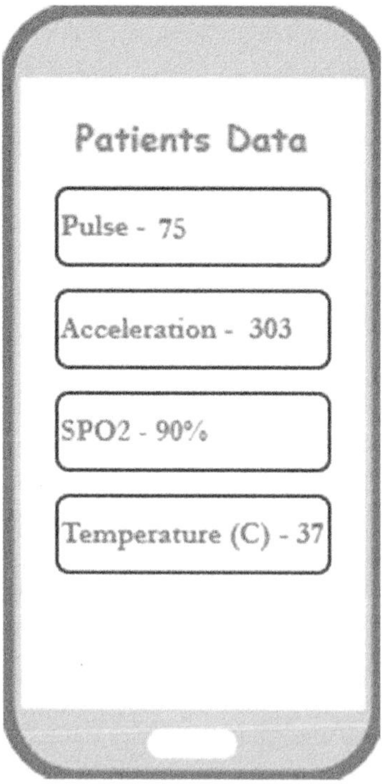

Figure 7.30 Patients data in Android application.

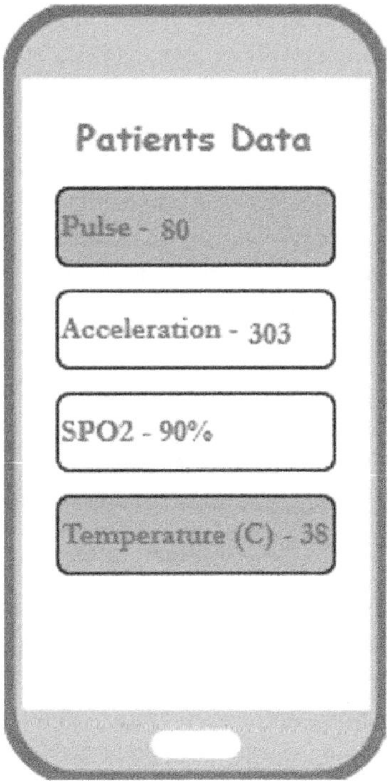

Figure 7.31 Patients data with alert.

monitor the patients before they reach the medical center. The device also can help to monitor older patients in their homes. The main use of the device is to monitor any patients or persons continually in real time from anywhere using the Android application and get vital information with closed-loop alerts so that immediate action can be taken to save patients' or others' lives in critical situations.

7.5 Conclusion and Future Work

7.5.1 Conclusion

In today's scenario, as advanced technology in innovation evolves quickly and rapidly, problems continue as technology continues to increase. In this paper, the various advanced approaches based on the patient health surveillance system presented by different authors in recent years have been discussed and studied. We have achieved that most SNW and IoT-based health surveillance systems for patients recognize the problem and problems associated with real-time data or information transfer and analysis.

The inspiration for working with the IoT and WSNs is having smart surveillance of patients, with a closed-loop alarm, plotting the real-time data in graph form, storing, sending the data to the cloud, and fetching the data in an Android application for monitoring. After completing the experiment, the final results were stored in the ThingSpeak cloud represented as a graph, and the data was sent to the Android application having a closed-loop. This technique was found easier and more reliable for sending real-time data to the cloud with the help of ThingSpeak. With the help of the D1 WeMos mini Wi-Fi module and the Arduino IDE, it was possible to send the real-time data wirelessly, directly to the cloud via ThingSpeak,. Finally, we proposed a patient-monitoring smart surveillance system based on WSNs and IoT, which can reliably analyze and efficiently monitor the collected data from the cloud in real-time within an Android application with closed loop.

7.5.2 Future Work

Future work includes widespread connection of monitoring devices in one application, application of machine learning algorithms to the stored data that have been saved in the cloud to automatically detect the patient's health, and connection of more vital sign sensors in the monitoring device to sense more parameters to help doctors.

References

1 Chen, H., Jia, X., and Li, H. (2011). A brief introduction to IoT gateway. In: *IET International Conference on Communication Technology and Application (ICCTA 2011)*, 610–613. IET.

2 Kim, J.S. (2015). The introduction of IoT (internet of things) technologies and policy directions. *Review of Korea Contents Association* 13 (1): 18–24.

3 Gokhale, P., Bhat, O., and Bhat, S. (2018). Introduction to IOT. *International Advanced Research Journal in Science, Engineering and Technology* 5 (1): 41–44.

4 Sanchez, L., Muñoz, L., Galache, J.A. et al. (2014). SmartSantander: IoT experimentation over a smart city testbed. *Computer Networks* 61: 217–238.

5 Lee, M., Hwang, J., and Yoe, H. (2013). Agricultural production system based on IoT. In: *2013 IEEE 16Th International Conference on Computational Science and Engineering*, 833–837. IEEE.

6 Lee, H., Lee, K., and Shin, Y. (2012). A GTS allocation scheme for emergency data transmission in cluster-tree WSNs. In: *2012 14th International Conference on Advanced Communication Technology (ICACT)*, 675–678. IEEE.

7 Singh, D.P., Bhateja, V., and Soni, S.K. (2013). An efficient cluster-based routing protocol for WSNs using time series prediction-based data reduction scheme. *International Journal of Measurement Technologies and Instrumentation Engineering (IJMTIE)* 3 (3): 18–34.
8 Xu, K., Wang, Q., Hassanein, H., and Takahara, G. (2005). Optimal wireless sensor networks (WSNs) deployment: minimum cost with lifetime constraint. In: *WiMob'2005, IEEE International Conference on Wireless and Mobile Computing, Networking and Communications*, vol. 3, 454–461. IEEE.
9 Luo, Z. (2012). Overview of applications of wireless sensor networks. *International Journal of Innovative Technology and Exploring Engineering* 1 (4): 4–6.
10 Zheng, L.I. and Shu-guang, M.I.A.O. (2010). Application of WSNs in mine laneway monitoring system based on ZigBee [J]. *Instrument Technique and Sensor*. https://en.cnki.com.cn/Article_en/CJFDTotal-YBJS201008020.htm.
11 Mpitziopoulos, A., Gavalas, D., Konstantopoulos, C., and Pantziou, G. (2009). A survey on jamming attacks and countermeasures in WSNs. *IEEE Communication Surveys and Tutorials* 11 (4): 42–56.
12 Bojanova, I. and Samba, A. (2011). Analysis of cloud computing delivery architecture models. In: *2011 IEEE Workshops of International Conference on Advanced Information Networking and Applications*, 453–458. IEEE.
13 Chi, Q., Yan, H., Zhang, C. et al. (2014). A reconfigurable smart sensor interface for industrial WSN in IoT environment. *IEEE Transactions on Industrial Informatics* 10 (2): 1417–1425.
14 Mitra, U., Emken, B.A., Lee, S. et al. (2012). KNOWME: a case study in wireless body area sensor network design. *IEEE Communications Magazine* 50 (5): 116–125.
15 Patel, S., Park, H., Bonato, P. et al. (2012). A review of wearable sensors and systems with application in rehabilitation. *Journal of Neuroengineering and Rehabilitation* 9 (1): 21.
16 Kothari, D., Thakker, M., Shah, V.A., and Gohel, T. (2013). A real time wireless multi-parameter monitoring system with ZigBee and LabVIEW. *International Journal of Current Engineering and Technology* 3 (5): 1667–1671.
17 Hackmann, G., Guo, W., Yan, G. et al. (2013). Cyber-physical codesign of distributed structural health monitoring with wireless sensor networks. *IEEE Transactions on Parallel and Distributed Systems* 25 (1): 63–72.
18 Misra, S., Chatterjee, S., and Obaidat, M.S. (2014). On theoretical modeling of sensor cloud: a paradigm shift from wireless sensor network. *IEEE Systems Journal* 11 (2): 1084–1093.
19 Simoes, N.A. and de Souza, G.B. (2016). A low cost automated data acquisition system for urban sites temperature and humidity monitoring

based in internet of things. In: *2016 1st International Symposium on Instrumentation Systems, Circuits and Transducers (INSCIT)*, 107–112. IEEE.

20 Zakaria, Y. and Michael, K. (2017). An integrated cloud-based wireless sensor network for monitoring industrial wastewater discharged into water sources. *Wireless Sensor Network* 9: 290–301.

21 Xie, G., Ota, K., Dong, M. et al. (2017). Energy-efficient routing for mobile data collectors in wireless sensor networks with obstacles. *Peer-to-Peer Networking and Applications* 10 (3): 472–483.

22 Vasisht, D., Kapetanovic, Z., Won, J. et al. (2017). Farmbeats: an iot platform for data-driven agriculture. In: *14th {USENIX} Symposium on Networked Systems Design and Implementation ({NSDI} 17)*, 515–529.

23 Miqdad, A., Kadir, K., and Ahmed, S.F. (2017). Development of data acquisition system for temperature and humidity monitoring scheme. In: *2017 IEEE 4th International Conference on Smart Instrumentation, Measurement and Application (ICSIMA)*, 1–4. IEEE.

24 AlSkaif, T., Bellalta, B., Zapata, M.G., and Ordinas, J.M.B. (2017). Energy efficiency of MAC protocols in low data rate wireless multimedia sensor networks: a comparative study. *Ad Hoc Networks* 56: 141–157.

25 Modieginyane, K.M., Letswamotse, B.B., Malekian, R., and Abu-Mahfouz, A.M. (2018). Software defined wireless sensor networks application opportunities for efficient network management: a survey. *Computers and Electrical Engineering* 66: 274–287.

26 Sethi, S. and Sahoo, R.K. (2019). Design of WSN in real time application of health monitoring system. In: *Virtual and Mobile Healthcare: Breakthroughs in Research and Practice*, 643–658. IGI Global.

27 Kaur, H., Atif, M., and Chauhan, R. (2020). An internet of healthcare things (IoHT)-based healthcare monitoring system. In: *Advances in Intelligent Computing and Communication*, 475–482. Singapore: Springer.

28 API request, https://thingspeak.com/channels/952366/api_keys, accessed on 01.12.2019 at 12.35 PM.

29 WeMos D1 mini - Mini NodeMcu 4M, https://www.amazon.in/gp/product/B07LCHS2MM/ref=ox_sc_act_title_1?smid=A3HAGIAPX2OISQ&psc=1, accessed on 01.12.2019 at 12.40 PM.

30 Arduino IDE, https://www.arduino.cc/en/Main/Software, accessed on 01.12.2019 at 12.45 PM.

31 ThingSpeak IoT platform, https://thingspeak.com, accessed on 01.12.2019 at 12.45 PM.

8

An IoMT-Based Smart Remote Monitoring System for Healthcare

Chetna Kaushal[1], Md Khairul Islam[2], Anshu Singla[1], and Md Al Amin[3]

[1] *Chitkara University Institute of Engineering and Technology, Chitkara University, Punjab, India*
[2] *Department of Information and Communication Technology, Islamic University, Kushtia, Bangladesh*
[3] *Department of Computer Science and Engineering, Prime University, Dhaka, Bangladesh*

8.1 Introduction

Cancer is a disorder where the body's cells grow rapidly creating a malignant tumor; cancers are called after the body part where they begin or continue to spread to the nearest body part (e.g., lung cancer). Cancer found in the cervix tissue is generally known as cervical cancer. The cervix act as an interface between the uterus and vagina [1].

Cervical intraepithelial neoplasia (CIN) is the unwanted growth of a woman's cervix. It makes the way to the cancer called cervical cancer, and this precancerous CIN can be divided into three grades (CIN-I, -II, and -III).

At the early stage of cervical cancer, no symptoms are commonly detected. Later signs can include frequent menstrual bleeding, stomach discomfort, or pain during periods or after menopause or sexual activity [1]. After sexual intercourse, pain is not a symptom, but postcoital bleeding can be a symptom of cervical cancer about to happen or present [2].

The main cause of cervical cancer is Human Papillomavirus infection (HPV). About 90% or cervical cancer cases have been confirmed to have been infected with HPV for a long period [3, 4]. Generally, HPV has moved from one human to another during sex. Thus, according to the Cleveland

IoT-Enabled Smart Healthcare Systems, Services and Applications, First Edition.
Edited by Shalli Rani, Maheswar Rajagopal, Neeraj Kumar and Syed Hassan Ahmed Shah.

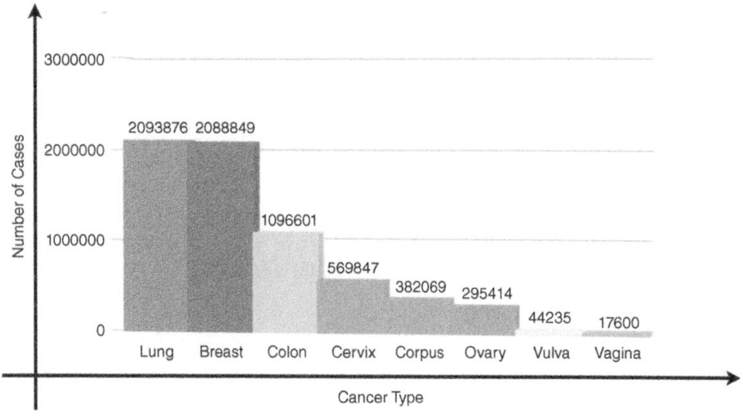

Figure 8.1 Different types of cancer cases found in the world in 2018.

Clinic, about 80% of people who are sexually active will carry HPV at any point in their lives, but it doesn't mean that every woman infected with HPV will be diagnosed with cervical cancer. [5, 6]. The risk of cervical cancer increases with alcohol consumption and smoking (which are important risk factors in all cancers), use of birth control pills for a long time (five or more years), and having multiple sexual partners at an early age. However, these are less significant risk factors [1, 7]. Cervical cancer is diagnosed in women above 30, and cancer cells require about 10–20 years to develop [6].

Figure 8.1 depicts different cancer cases found, based on a 2018 report. Lung, breast, colon, and cervix are the top four. Lung cancer cases reported worldwide are almost 2.1 million with 85% mortality, and it stands on the top of the table. Breast and colon cancers reported on 2018 are 2 million and 1.1 million cases, respectively. Mortality of breast and colon cancer are almost 30% and 50%, respectively. Cervical cancer is the world's fourth most common cancer [8, 9] and the fourth most prominent in women [10]. Nearly 529 000 patients were diagnosed in 2012, which is nearly 8% of the estimated cancer cases [6]; its mortality rate is 50.4%.

Figure 8.2 depicts the cervical cancer cases and deaths of each country based on the Human Development Index (HDI). HDI is defined by education, per capita income, and other indices. Thus, countries with medium HDI have most of the cases and deaths, but countries with very high HDI have comparatively very few cases and deaths. Dramatically, cervical cancer cases in low HDI countries are similar to those in very high HDI countries, but death cases are high [8]. According to the World Health Organization (WHO), developed countries reported approximately 70% of cervical cancers and 90% of deaths [66]. In 2018, about 570 000 women were diagnosed, and almost 54.57% of the patients died, according to the WHO report.

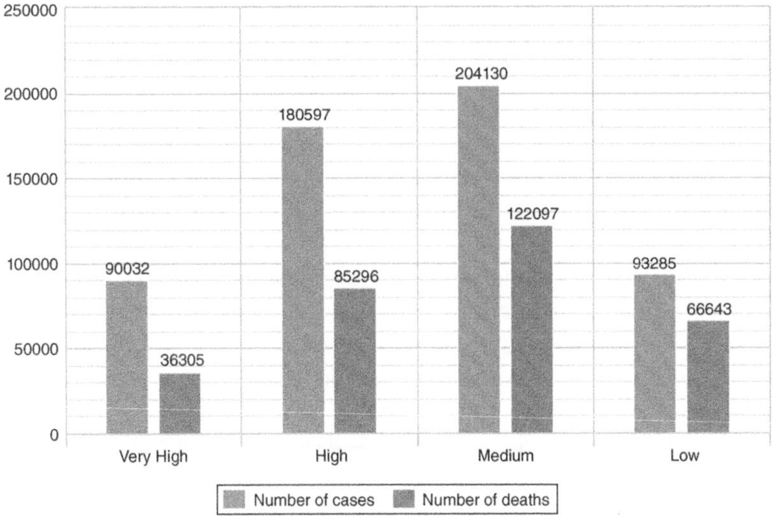

Figure 8.2 Cervical cancer cases and deaths depending on the HDI value of countries.

Although death rates have increased by 4% in recent times, developed countries have reduced their death rates in large numbers. However, women from 42 underdeveloped countries are most likely affected by cervical cancer [11]. About 84% of cases and 88% of deaths have been recorded in underdeveloped countries [8]. Squamous cell carcinoma (80%), adenocarcinoma (15%), adenosquamous carcinoma (3–5%), small cell carcinoma, and neuroendocrine cancer are the most frequent forms of cervical cancer [9].

Due to the extreme death rate, many methods have been developed to identify pre-stage of cervical cancer so that the chances of survival can be improved by early diagnosis and early treatment of cervix cells. Different computer-aided screening methods are used to detect an infected cervix before it has transformed into an invasive cancer. This computer-assisted diagnosis (CAD) system is common, simple to use, and less time-consuming. The Pap test (Pap smear), liquid-based cytology (LBC), HPV DNA checking, visual inspection, and visual analysis of acetic acid are different screening procedures discussed in the literature [12].

For the past 50 years, the Pap test has lowered the case and death rate of cervical cancer in the US [9, 12]. The Pap test demanded a high amount of test capital, which has limited its use in developing countries. In the Pap test with conventional cytology, the cells are carefully scratched out of the ectocervix and endocervix by trained, skilled pathologists with a spatula or brush and smeared under a microscope slide [12]. It has a relatively low sensitivity of 54% but a high precision of 94%[13].

In LBC, cells are obtained in an identical method to a conventional Pap test. Samples are smeared into a liquid of maintained space. After filters or centrifuges, the sample is passed to a slide. It is a procedure that is more costly than traditional cytology and requires extra resources and expensive tools. No difference in relative sensitivity and precision from the traditional way was found in LBC, but there is a benefit in evaluating high-risk HPV in the cervix cells. Moreover, in LBC, proper sample selection is not feasible [12, 14].

Automated Pap analysis helps to minimize errors by analyzing Pap smear slides using the CAD tool. AutoPap and AutoCyte Screen are two automatic Pap types. In AutoPap, centered on an algorithm, the sample of the slide is checked and graded. While it does not explain which of the cells is irregular, it may describe the cervix's actual condition [15].

Methods for visual screening are easy and can be carried out by a professional doctor or nurse, are comparatively cheap, do not require laboratory space, and have instant results. The different visual analysis types are as follows: unaided visual inspection and visual inspection with acetic acid (VIA) treatment. It is a representation of the cervix without acetic acid in the human eye. This reveals bad performance [16–18].

To identify pre-cancerous lesions, visual inspection after application of 3–5% acetic acid is performed. It can also be identified with the human eye, known as cervicoscopy, or immediate visual inspection. Changeable coagulation of cellular proteins is caused by applying 3–5% acetic acid and invasive cancer regions containing a significant number of the same cells in the epithelial cells [19, 20]. In order to correctly detect pre-cancerous lesions, VIA could do better than the Pap test [21]. Between 45% and 79% of women at high risk of developing cervical cancer have been correctly detected by qualified doctors and mid-level providers [22]. VIA indicates higher false-positive cases than the Pap approach.

However, it is hard to find professional pathologists to identify pre-cancerous cervix cells by the naked eye. Community and researchers developed Internet of Things- (IoT-) [23] and Internet of Healthcare Things- (IoHT-) [24] based devices for pre-screening. IoHT-based devices work for Pap-smear images and classify normal and abnormal images only. But there is a need of a system where women can have pre-screening of cervical cancer at low cost with timely accurate diagnosis. The major challenge in such implementation requires computer vision and computational resources along with knowledge of medical sciences. Low resource and cost-effective settings are required with highly secured and confidential data for preliminary screening tests. If the test results are positive, then the patient may be recommended or referred for colposcopy and further treatment with expert doctors. This preliminary screening may help the patient in reducing the chances of cervical cancer and can be treated by midwives and nurses. This may reduce the burden on the experts and may help the patient in early diagnosis.

Colposcopy or CIN images of the patients are hard to get but Intel and MobileODT through a competition on Kaggle in 2017 classified different types of cervix to detect the precancerous conditions of patients [25].

With continued improvement in screening methods and HPV vaccination programs in developed countries, the disparity of burden between developed countries and women in resource-poor settings becomes even more profound. Nearly 85% of cervical cancer deaths occur in low- and middle-income-countries, and cervical cancer is a leading cause of cancer death in women in the developing world. If women are timely screened once after the age of 35 years, there is a 70% reduction in the risk of death due to cervical cancer. This can also reduce the disparity among women in developed countries and developing countries. The sentiments of women in developing countries may be hurt while to undergo physical examination. The women's hesitant nature gives us a high need to have a portable, wireless, and confidential device to have pre-screening by midwives, nearby healthcare centers, or by themselves. The persistent HPV infection may lead to cervix cancer. The timely pre-screening may define the important determinants and timely clearance with small treatments, which further reduces the viral persistence that may lead to cervical cancer. Recent image capturing technology can be used to make a portable, low-cost, wireless, and confidential device that can be easily accessed and used by nearby healthcare centers.

8.2 Literature Review

IoT technology is an evolving healthcare field that has decreased patient waiting time and ensures treatment quality, even at home, by automating real-time procedures. Various medical imaging experiments have been performed using IoT, known as Internet of Medical Things (IoMT), to pave the way for automation approaches.

He et al. explore cancer diagnostic approaches using deep learning algorithms such as convolutional neural networks (CNNs) and autoencoders (AE) [65]. To detect cancer, images of multiple organs or cells are used (such as lung, colon, breast, cervical). Various pre-trained models such as VGG16, ResNet, and GoogleNet are used to distinguish between benign and malignant breast cells [26]. These pre-trained models used average pooling and are attached to a completely connected layer. In a study [27], first of all Pap smear images were taken of the cervical cells from the Herlev data set. Then they introduced random forest (a machine learning algorithm) to classify normal and abnormal images. They extracted features depending on weight and used a 10-fold cross-validation for training. A custom CNN model called CXNN for classification has been created by Sun et al. [27]. They tuned optimization and training hyperparameters for CXNN.

Lu and Liu [28] explain clinical treatment and remote monitoring of ECG in real-time using IoT in medical science. While they offer the concept of integrating IoT in healthcare, they do not explain IoT devices or how they are linked. In Ijaz et al. [29], a hybrid prediction model (HPM) is employed to provide early prediction of type 2 diabetes and hypertension using machine learning algorithms. The HPM of the analysis can be implemented using the IoMT, which stores evaluated risk factors on a safe remote server and provides the patient with the proper course. The authors suggest an IoT-based android app for future work but don't explain how data is gathered by the sensor and linked to the mobile app. For future work, they suggest an IoT-based android app, but they do not explain how the sensor captures or links information to the app. Rahman et al. [30] describe how the diagnosed cancer patients should maintain a secure routine during treatment. However, covering patients' daily lives is difficult, so many IoT-based models have been developed to obtain a real-time report of patients' conditions and activities. This study shows the identification of the state of the skeletons and the exercise of cancer patients; however, how this addresses cancer patients' issues is unclear. An IoT network system employed in Onasanya and Elshakankiri [23] mainly focuses on the wireless topology of different devices for diagnosis, recovery, and patient management. It is done by the analysis of health data obtained by IoT network systems and other mobile devices to help health professionals and make urgent assessments on cancer conditions.

Chandy [31] discusses IoT integration for multiple diagnostic systems of medical imaging such as MRI, x-rays, CT, and ultrasound. However, there is still a need for further work on encryption algorithms to have a secure IoT medical device so as to avoid any misuse of data. Onasanya and Elshakankiri [32] created a smart healthcare infrastructure, especially for patients with cancer. They divided their entire solution into five-layer approaches and joined them to construct an efficient, interconnected IoT framework. Specifically, these layers are a service layer for identification, tracking, and follow-up, a data center layer for capturing cancer patient data, a cancer treatment layer for visualizing patient reports, a hospital layer for moving patient status to a doctor or nurse, and a protection layer for preventing unexpected hospital incidents.

Single-board computers are developed by Parra et al. [33] to offer a low-cost diagnosis for underdeveloped countries using a Raspberry Pi (RP) computer. They have developed two devices to diagnose cervix cell before turning into invasive cancer with real-time results. One is based on visual inspection of the cervix's nuclei high-resolution image implemented by IoT devices with deep learning algorithms for classifying cervix cells named PiHRME. Moreover, another molecular level test of cervical cells is also implemented by IoT to identify cells' current condition, called PiReader. Both are easy to use and cost half of the previous manual approaches. Although it is cost-effective to use the Raspberry Pi computer, it can't be used to store and train with a lot of images. Khamparia et al. [24] employ the IoHT for the classification of cervical cell images collected from a Pap-dating approach. In order to accomplish the mission, they have merged both IoT and image classification algorithms. To distinguish images, they use both machine learning and deep learning algorithms. Transfer learning was also used to reuse the pre-developed knowledge of models. They claim a 97% accuracy because the data set is very limited, which causes the trained model to be overfitted. Cervical cancer screening will need a huge data set to train a robust model, which is still a concern for researchers.

8.3 Methodology

8.3.1 IoT Device for Image Acquisition

In this part, we describe an IoT-based cervix detection healthcare system. We have used a Raspberry Pi (RP) board in the device, with a Raspberry Pi camera and an ultrasonic sensor. Robotics equipment is used in the device, which open the labia minora (LM). A labia minora and cervix detection algorithm is implemented in that RP board for capturing the correct organs. At first, the camera will take a photo to find the labia minora because it is the front part of cervix. After capturing the photo, the algorithm will detect the position of the labia minora (LM). After fixing the position of LM, it will be treated as an object. Then we will use ultrasonic sensor to measure the distance from the sensor to LM. We will measure the distance in order to correctly open the vagina by using the medical equipment, which will come from the IoT device, and it will work automatically, without any needed assistance. So if the equipment doesn't get accurate measure and location, then it will not be able to open the vagina. After opening the vagina, the camera will take a photo of the cervix. Then, the algorithm will work to

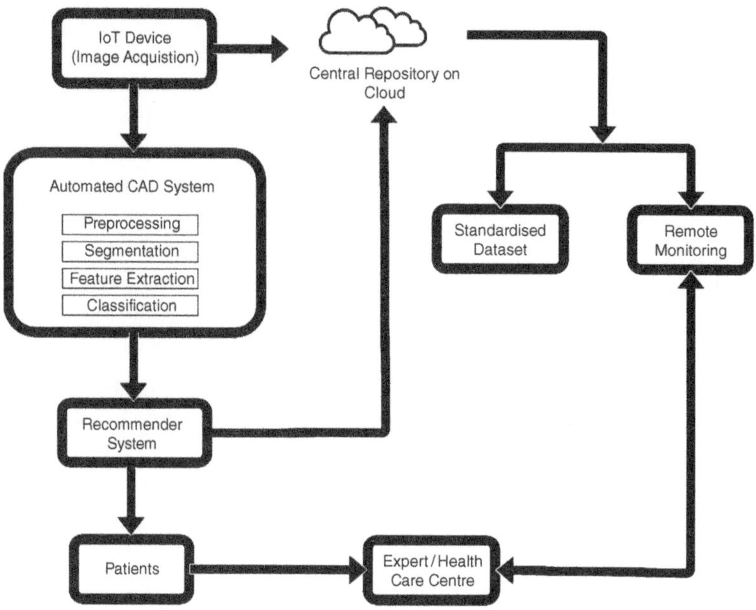

Figure 8.3 Proposed methodology for IoMT-based smart remote monitoring system for cervix cancer.

detect cervix precancerous condition automatically. Figure 8.3 describes the total communication processes of IoT device elements with proper direction and command. The following subsections describe all the devices, step by step.

8.3.1.1 Raspberry Pi

In the United Kingdom, the RP foundation developed RP, which is a series of small single-board computers launched in 2012. It is known as minicomputer, which performs computational processes. It is widely used for real-time image or video processing, IoT-based applications, and robotics-based applications. In this board, we can add a camera, a sensor to measure distance, and other important devices. The Raspberry Pi includes a 1.2 GHz quad-core 1.4 GHz, 1 GB RAM, the Broadcom SoC, GPU, built-in Wi-Fi and Bluetooth 4.0, and 10/100 Mbps Ethernet. Most people use it to build hardware projects, to make home automation, to process algorithms, and so on [34, 35]. As of 2016, about eight million Raspberry Pi had been sold, and it is projected to be one the most popular single-board computers in the world [36]. We have implemented RP to detect and open the labia minora and at last detect the cervix using a pretrained model in the board (Figure 8.4).

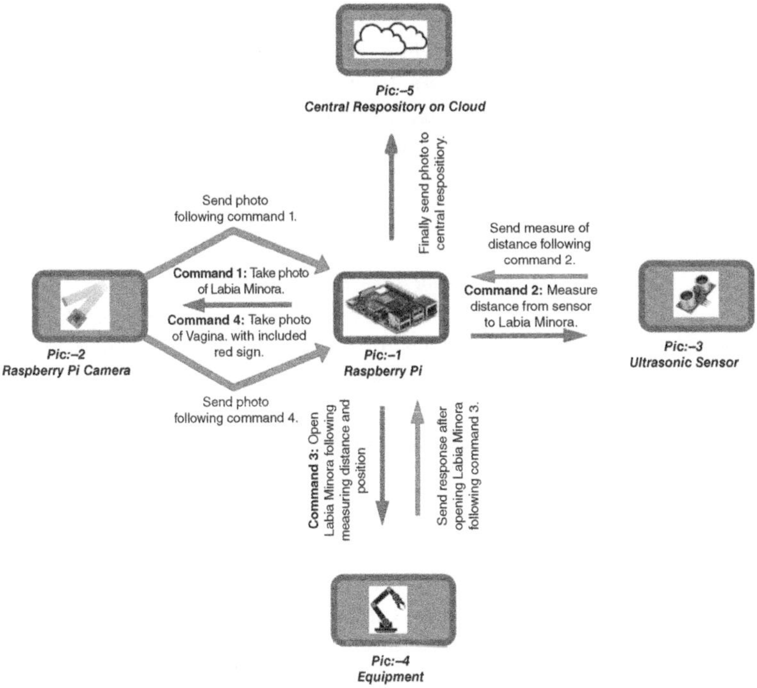

Figure 8.4 Automated IoT-based image acquisition process.

Camera: Raspberry Pi has an embedded camera module (version 2). It has a Sony IMX219 eight megapixel camera sensor, and it's able to deliver almost five-megapixel resolution of image or 1080p high-definition video at 30 frames per second and still shots up to 2592×1944 resolution. Time lapse, slow motion video, IP CCTV and monitoring, and more are included in this module. The camera module was attached to a Raspberry Pi by a 15 pin ribbon cable and to the dedicated 15 pin MIPI camera serial interface, which was designed for interfacing to cameras and has a BCM2835 processor [37, 38].

8.3.1.2 Sensor

The ultrasonic sensor HC-SR04 is used to measure the distance of an object from the sensor. This sensor is able to measure distances from 2 mm (0.02 m) to 400 cm (4 m). This sensor is the most popular sensor used in many applications and devices where we need to measure distances. Put another way, we can say an ultrasonic sensor is an electronic device that measures distances by emitting ultrasonic sound waves and convert this waves into an electrical signal. It is generally used with microcontroller and microprocessor platforms such as Arduino, ARM, PIC, and Raspberry Pi. Ultrasonic sensors are used in IoT- and robotic-based platforms for detecting the targeted object, as well as in manufacturing technologies. Notably, ultrasonic technology has enabled in the medical sector or health sector to produce images of internal organs, to detect tumors, and to ensure the health of babies in the womb [39]. Now, we can use an ultrasonic sensor with RP [40]. RP works at 3.3 V logic, but the ultrasonic sensor HC-SR04 works at 5 V. Thus, if we want to connect the ultrasonic sensor with this RP, then we have to connect an echo pin to RP before connecting it to the sensor. At first we have to connect the trig pin of the ultrasonic sensor with the physical pin GPIO23 of the RP. Then we have to use a combination of 680 Ω and 1.5 kΩ resistor for converting the echo pin to 3.3 V logic. And we need to connect it to a physical pin GPIO24 of the RP. Then the problem will be solved. Finally we have to write programming algorithms on Raspberry Pi to enable and perform the required task by the ultrasonic sensor.

8.3.1.3 Equipment

The IoT- and robotics-based equipment used will be able to close or open the vagina carefully as it is a very sensitive organ of women. The equipment can move left, right, up, and down using the direction from RP. RP is directed by using the data of the sensor and algorithmic calculations.

After taking photos of the cervix, the device will store the image, storage embedded on RP board, and finally a trained machine learning algorithm will produce the desired diagnosis for cervical cancer. This algorithm will be implemented in the Raspberry Pi board to classify the cervix type using the image. Now this result and image will be sent to a cloud repository from RP storage with regard to the result about the patient. We have to install a cloud repository app using an Internet connection to the RP board. For details, see Doshi et al. [41] Finally the result and corresponding data is stored for both patient and the health team's supervision.

8.3.2 Central Repository

The CAD system is an IoT-based healthcare system that can be used at home without going to the hospital to check for cervical cancer conditions. After checking the results, the CAD system saves the corresponding images from each patient to the central cloud archive for further use by the research institute and others. In addition to the classifiers, the efficiency of the classifiers is strongly dependent on the number of images/data points. The central repository is linked to a healthcare data center through a server. In order to gain insight into the data, central repository data can be analyzed, synchronized, and grouped. Researchers can also build their model more robustly and reliably by using repository data to improve the CAD system's adaptability. As we intend to share the central archive for public use, we can recheck the records so that there is no violation of patient confidentiality. We should follow the government's rules and regulations for setting up certain networks and equipment. And patients should also know the guidelines and policies of the CAD system [23].

8.3.3 Automatic Computer Assisted Diagnosis (ACAD)

Very few specialist pathologists are capable of identifying pre-cancer lesions using a visual inspection process. Expert availability and their attitude have an effect on proper identification. CAD is an emerging approach that will provide the pathologist with advantages of fast results, higher accuracy, and reduced time and suffering of patients. In medical imaging, the use of CAD in the study of cytological images of cervix lesions has become a topic of interest.

8.3.3.1 Preprocessing

IoT devices use sensors to capture images of the targeted area. Now these images have to be extracted to collect information from them. So we can do segmentation and image extraction of features. But we have to preprocess the data before getting to this point because due to the atmosphere or other factors, the image of the IoT system can be distorted or can contain noise [42].

Unexpected occurrences, such as noise, outliers, and missing pixel values, may have a major effect on segmentation efficiency, feature extraction, and model classification. So we will preprocess the images captured by the IoT network before storing the images in the central repository. It is possible to categorize image preprocessing in medical imaging into four parts. The first one concerns the correction of pixel brightness, also known as the transformation of brightness. After brightness corrections, the output pixel values of the image are strongly dependent on the input pixel values of the images. Contrast modifications are one of the key components of preprocessing, especially in medical imaging. It is possible to break brightness corrections into two grayscale and brightness transformation sections. Grayscale is commonly used in medical imaging, especially in the detection of cell levels.

Second, geometric transition restores the position of the pixel, which is usually distorted by the external environment, such as blurred transformation of images. This phase of the technique involves rotation, translation, shear, and scale. Such preprocessing methods are often used for increasing images database to balance the data set of different labels.

Third, filter the image to retrieve critical information using certain kernels that improve or smooth the edge condition. As a result, the models are able to learn the necessary knowledge

Fourth, restoration of the image, which entails improving the deteriorated images. Most of the image loss occurs due to temperature, camera lens, or miscommunication of the electro-optical sensor. Two methods of restoration are available: deterministic and stochastic; both are important for medical imaging tasks. The first is used where noise and other deterioration are known. The second one works depending on a small group of pre-enhanced images position and restoration [43]. There should be no loss of information, patches, lesions if any i.e. affected area during preprocessing of image.

8.3.3.2 Segmentation

In order to complete the purpose, image segmentation is one of the essential tasks. Segmentation of the image helps to distinguish and differentiate the appropriate organs and cells from other undesirable areas; in a nutshell, it identifies the most significant area that includes the majority of the information referred to as the region of interest (ROI). Image segmentation is an automated ROI separation method that takes into account that the region does not overlap with the embedded correlative portion. The method of image segmentation in medical imaging is managed and implemented by supervised and unsupervised algorithms. Picture segmentation typically operates on two-dimensional images, but it has now been applied using a co-evolutionary kernel on three-dimensional MRI images [44, 45].

Different methods of segmentation are discussed in the following subsections to classify the cervix area of interest for visual inspection:

8.3.3.2.1 Clustering Clustering is an unsupervised ROI segmentation approach that aims to locate a pixel space of the same or near intensity. It can work with fewer data and needs no particular labeling of the training data since it is unsupervised. For segmentation, there are several clustering algorithms such as k-means, fuzzy c-means, and hard c-means. Among them, one of the most used and best-performing algorithms is k-means. For any label, it finds an average mean intensity. It calculates the mean intensity of each pixel, and if the mean of each pixel is near the individual label, that pixel is assigned to that label space [46]. In Bai et al. [47], ROI segmentation was performed on HSV images using the k-means algorithm. Here, first, histogram-based thresholding is applied to eliminate the image's mirror effect if it appears. Then the images are converted from RGB to HSV images, and the ROI is found based on the image's V space using k-means.

8.3.3.2.2 Region Growing The region growing (RG) algorithm is a semiautomated base segmentation technique. It considers the correlative region on the basis of certain previously established parameters (e.g., edge or intensity). And it needs to refer to a region from which the correlative field is detected, which is why it is semiautomated. It keeps adding areas until the criteria are not fulfilled. On a grayscale picture, it performs well. It converts the images to HSI space first and then adds RG to separate ROI They used this algorithm on 111 cervical cancer screening photos, [48].

8.3.3.2.3 Threshold Threshold is a threshold-based segmentation method where a label is given an intensity greater than the threshold value and another label is assigned to the items where the value is less than the threshold. It is usually a segmentation of two labels, but multithresholding is feasible.

8.3.3.2.4 Artificial Neural Network It is one of the most used segmentation methods, but learning is ultimately supervised. It is used to segment the training data set with weights and other parameters specified so that information loss is low. It can then segment the ROI from the test/new data set image.

Segmentation methods vary much depending on the image domain. But an inaccurate segmentation technique selection can be the cause of a loss of information. Thus, the selection of an image segmentation technique will help increase the accuracy of any project.

8.3.3.3 Feature Extraction and Selection

Features are extracted and selected before classifier models are implemented. The efficiency of the model classifiers is strongly dependent on the extraction and selection techniques of the features. The classifier's model results may not be satisfactory due to existing noise and multiple features. Feature extraction and selection techniques lower computing time and memory requirements while also improving the performance of classifiers. [49]. We had to extract features from images of cervix cells first based on morphology, texture, and intensity. In medical imaging, there are many feature extraction techniques that are used. Some of the most used extraction techniques are discussed here:

8.3.3.3.1 Morphological Feature Extraction The extraction of features is known as morphological feature extraction, based on the size and shape of artifacts [50]. Size and shape are expressed as a mathematical value. In contrast to the standard cervix cell, an increase in the size of cervix cells, which is measured and viewed as a function. And the shape of cervix cells, such as round, invasive, or smooth, is often taken as a feature. Various methods are used to assess the size and form of cells from images such as threshold, clustering, and statistical techniques. Morphological-based feature extraction has been used by many researchers [51–54].

8.3.3.3.2 Texture Based Feature Extraction A low-level feature of the images is the texture. In the case of morphological (size and shape) and intensity-(color-) based features, it may be the same for two objects. But in order to distinguish these two things, we need to consider the smoothness or the coarseness, or the continuity of colors (texture feature). Thus, the extraction of the texture attribute is the nonlinear, semantic, or regional level/position of the brightness of color in the images. There are several methods for estimating texture features, such as the gray level co-occurrence matrix and the wavelet transform. There are several pieces of cervical cancer screening studies that have used extraction of the texture-based element [50, 55–58].

8.3.3.3.3 Intensity Based Feature Extraction The intensity-based feature is the extraction of information using the color distribution from gray or color images. But the continuity or smoothness of the edge of the image and other areas is not considered in this category of feature extraction. The strength base attribute was used in cervical cancer screening problems to learn and identify the multiple cervix lesion disorders [50, 59, 60].

We need to select features after extracting the attributes so that the classifier works well for unseen images and is robust. Yet in supervised learning there are numerous methods for feature selection, such as unsupervised basic learning, which uses the correlation for the collection of features; decision tree algorithms; information gain; and dimension reduction techniques (PCA) [50, 61–63].

8.3.3.4 Classification Model

The data set contains three types of CIN: high-grade CIN, low-grade CIN, and normal cervix. Thus, we need to identify the various conditions of the cervix using the extracted and chosen features of the images. We need classifiers to classify between various targets or labels. Hence, based on the correlation to the target, classifiers are used to distinguish each image between targets. It may be supervised or unsupervised by classifiers. Various researchers have used various machine learning algorithms to detect high, low-grade CIN, or normal cervix (classifier). But the most popular algorithms for machine learning are linear regression, logistic regression, decision tree, SVM, naive Bayes, k-nearest neighbors, random forest, and XGBoost, among others. Mariarputham and Stephen [49] have used SVM to classify Pap smear images into seven target labels. Lu et al. [64] have deployed five different machine learning algorithms for cervical cancer diagnosis.

We need an assessment metric to measure the efficiency of the classifiers. The CAD framework must work well enough that the shortage of experts may be compensated. There are several metrics for measurement, such as accuracy, sensitivity, and specificity. The total number of true positive and true negative points against the total target points is determined by the accuracy. The sensitivity indicates the percentage of patients at risk of being affected, and the specificity determines the percentage of patients not at risk. Thus, we can measure the success of the CAD system based on these metrics. Generally, performance tests on unseen (test) data and the model trained on the data set are overfitting or underfitting.

8.3.4 Recommender System

We use the central cloud repository to store the latest image of the cervix's lesions situation and the outcome. This will be passed to the healthcare staff to recommend certain procedures to be followed. Women are generally concerned about their health in developed countries. However, in underdeveloped areas, it is nearly impossible to keep track of their health status on a regular basis. To reduce the disparity and help women in underdeveloped countries, the proposed IoMT-based healthcare system will help them to connect to the medical team even from home. The health services will consider using their data from the central database if any situation arises and suggest going to the hospital for recheck-up or treatment. Even the medical staff will inform the doctor or pathologists in the available time so that no miscommunication occurs. This entire procedure not only benefits people with difficulties in developing countries but also helps women in developed countries to save time.

8.4 Use Case of Real-Time Remote Monitoring System

The major challenges in the area of real-time applications of healthcare is privacy, scalability, and compliance to transfer patients' data from one to another network. Another major challenge for IoMT is to allocate resources

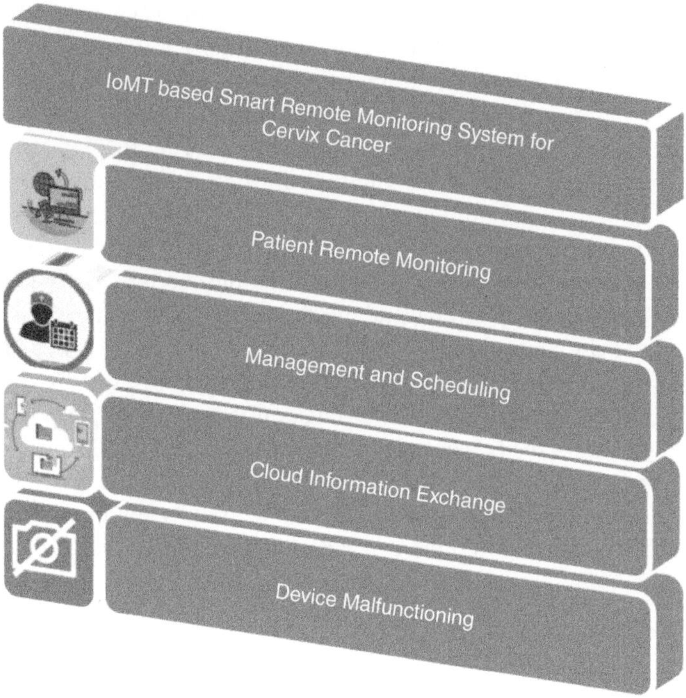

Figure 8.5 An IoMT-based smart remote monitoring system for cervix cancer.

such as doctors and midwives to the patient immediately and locate everything using tracking devices. Cloud storage of a cervical cancer patient data must have the following features (Figure 8.5).

8.4.1 Patient Remote Monitoring

Immediate availability of doctors, nurses, and a nearby healthcare center is checked by IoMT using databases on the cloud. The connected devices on the cloud will be analyzed based on which monitoring schedules and efficient utilization of equipment will be maintained. Staff scheduling and resource allocation schemes will ensure the resource provision in right time and place, thereby reducing resource conflicts.

8.4.2 Management and Scheduling

A patient registers by visiting a nearby healthcare center or through a personal device registered on IoMT. As soon as a patient joins the network, she can be detected by the controller of the system, for example a software-defined networking (SDN) controller. The controller provides the features such as security, scalability, and flexibility to transfer the patient's data to cloud storage. The controller will also create a virtual network to maintain patient confidentiality. Patient monitoring from remote areas requires stable communication to acquire images either through wired or wireless networks. A doctor is assigned/allocated based on the availability. Follow-up schedules, diagnoses, and reports are sent to concerned parties through a management and scheduling subsystem.

8.4.3 Cloud Information Exchange

The data can be obtained from different remote locations and need to be shared among patients, doctors, midwives, and laboratories. Hospitals are the main center for data generation related to diagnosis and medical reports/records of patients. The data may be shared among heterogeneous environments: network to network, machine to network, cloud to single machine, or vice versa.

8.4.4 Device Malfunctioning

IoMT system will also monitor and generate an alert signal for connected medical devices when a device is malfunctioning. Receiving the malfunctioning indication for a device, medical staff will be allocated to take precautions and fix the equipment quickly, minimizing or even avoiding its downtime. In case the device connected malfunctions, the patient data will be transferred to the nearest center for monitoring. The remote monitoring of a patient can also help in tracking patients' health and timely instructions for the next course of action. Also, the in-time notification will help to fix the bugs of equipment before it is damaged beyond repair.

8.5 Conclusion

In the current scenario, we require a reasonable trade-off between the burden and benefits of screening. Cytology tests and colposcopies increase the burden at both ends: patient as well as experts. Thus, preliminary diagnosis may help women with the recommendation whether they should go for colposcopy or not. Apart from this, it may help to take care of women's sentiments by providing an automated low-cost, secured, and portable device in nearby healthcare centers which can be handled by midwives. The recommender system in the proposed methodology may help the patient with the appropriate advice for screening intervals if required and future actions to reduce incidence rate. If CIN I is diagnosed in the patient, the standard treatment of recommendation includes monitoring for progression and may reduce the incidence of CIN II and III with help of remote monitoring. Many developing countries have no cervical cancer screening programs due to lack of medical professionals and other resources. The proposed methodology will help the government and policy makers to have cervical cancer awareness programs, which will help in reducing the incidence of cervical cancer.

References

1 PDQ Screening and Prevention Editorial Board. Cervical cancer screening (pdq®): Patient version. *PDQ Cancer Information Summaries [Internet]*, 2002.

2 Tarney, C.M. and Han, J. (2014). Postcoital bleeding: a review on etiology, diagnosis, and management. *Obstetrics and Gynecology International* 2014.

3 Holland, J.F. and Pollock, R.E. (2010). *Holland-Frei Cancer Medicine*, vol. 8. PMPH-USA.

4 Kumar, V., Abbas, A.K., Fausto, N., and Mitchell, R.N. (2007). Cervical cancer. In: *Robbins Basic Pathology*, vol. *8*, 718–721. Saunders Elsevier.

5 Dunne, E.F. and Park, I.U. (2013). HPV and HPV-associated diseases. *Infectious Disease Clinics* 27 (4): 765–778.

6 Stewart, B.W. and Wild C.P. (2014). World cancer report 2014. *World Health Organization.*

7 National Cancer Institute (2016). Cervical cancer treatment (pdq®)–health professional version.

8 Arbyn, M., Weiderpass, E., Bruni, L. et al. (2020). Estimates of incidence and mortality of cervical cancer in 2018: a worldwide analysis. *The Lancet Global Health* 8 (2): e191–e203.

9 Jemal, A., Siegel, R., and Ward, E. (2007). Cervical cancer. *CA: A Cancer Journal for Clinicians* 57: 43–66.

10 Canavan, T.P. and Doshi, N.R. (2000). Cervical cancer. *American Family Physician* 61 (5): 1369–1376.

11 Canfell, K., Kim, J.J., Brisson, M. et al. (2020). Mortality impact of achieving who cervical cancer elimination targets: a comparative modelling analysis in 78 low-income and lower-middle-income countries. *The Lancet* 395 (10224): 591–603.

12 Mishra, G.A., Pimple, S.A., and Shastri, S.S. (2011). An overview of prevention and early detection of cervical cancers. *Indian Journal of Medical and Paediatric Oncology: Official Journal of Indian Society of Medical & Paediatric Oncology* 320 (3): 125.

13 Coste, J., Cochand-Priollet, B., de Cremoux, P. et al. (2003). Cross sectional study of conventional cervical smear, monolayer cytology, and human papillomavirus DNA testing for cervical cancer screening. *BMJ* 326 (7392): 733.

14 Ronco, G., Cuzick, J., Pierotti, P. et al. (2007). Accuracy of liquid based versus conventional cytology: overall results of new technologies for cervical cancer screening: randomised controlled trial. *BMJ* 335 (7609): 28.

15 Apgar, B.S. (2001). New tests for cervical cancer screening. *American Family Physician* 64 (5): 729.

16 Nene, B.M., Deshpande, S., Jayant, K. et al. (1996). Early detection of cervical cancer by visual inspection: a population-based study in rural India. *International Journal of Cancer* 68 (6): 770–773.

17 Singh, V., Sehgal, A., and Luthra, U.K. (1992). Screening for cervical cancer by direct inspection. *British Medical Journal* 304 (6826): 534–535.

18 Wesley, R., Sankaranarayanan, R., Mathew, B. et al. (1997). Evaluation of visual inspection as a screening test for cervical cancer. *British Journal of Cancer* 75 (3): 436–440.

19 Sankaranarayanan, R., Basu, P., Wesley, R.S. et al. (2004). Accuracy of visual screening for cervical neoplasia: results from an iarc multicentre study in India and Africa. *International Journal of Cancer* 110 (6): 907–913.

20 University of Zimbabwe and JHPIEGO Cervical Cancer Project (1999). Visual inspection with acetic acid for cervical-cancer screening: test qualities in a primary-care setting. *The Lancet* 353 (9156): 869–873.

21 Sherris, J., Wittet, S., Kleine, A. et al. (2009). Evidence-based, alternative cervical cancer screening approaches in low-resource settings. *International Perspectives on Sexual and Reproductive Health* 35 (3): 147–152.

22 Sankaranarayanan, R., Gaffikin, L., Jacob, M. et al. (2005). A critical assessment of screening methods for cervical neoplasia. *International Journal of Gynecology & Obstetrics* 89: S4–S12.

23 Onasanya, A. and Elshakankiri, M. (2017). Iot implementation for cancer care and business analytics/cloud services in healthcare systems. In: *Proceedings of the10th International Conference on Utility and Cloud Computing*, 205–206.

24 Khamparia, A., Gupta, D., de Albuquerque, V.H.C. et al. (2020). Internet of health things-driven deep learning system for detection and classification of cervical cells using transfer learning. *The Journal of Supercomputing*: 1–19.

25 Intel Kaggle (2017). Mobileodt cervical cancer screening, 2019.

26 Khan, S.U., Islam, N., Jan, Z. et al. (2019). A novel deep learning based framework for the detection and classification of breast cancer using transfer learning. *Pattern Recognition Letters* 125: 1–6.

27 Sun, G., Li, S., Cao, Y., and Lang, F. (2017). Cervical cancer diagnosis based on random forest. *International Journal of Performability Engineering* 13 (4).

28 Lu, D. and Liu, T. (2011). The application of iot in medical system. In: *2011 IEEE International Symposium on IT in Medicine and Education*, vol. 1, 272–275. IEEE.

29 Ijaz, M.F., Alfian, G., Syafrudin, M., and Rhee, J. (2018). Hybrid prediction model for type 2 diabetes and hypertension using dbscan-based outlier detection, synthetic minority over sampling technique (smote), and random forest. *Applied Sciences* 8 (8): 1325.

30 Rahman, A., Rashid, M., Le Kernec, J. et al. (2019). A secure occupational therapy framework for monitoring cancer patients' quality of life. *Sensors* 19 (23): 5258.

31 Chandy, A. (2019). A review on IoT based medical imaging technology for healthcare applications. *Journal of Innovative Image Processing (JIIP)* 1 (01): 51–60.

32 Onasanya, A. and Elshakankiri, M. (2019). Smart integrated iot healthcare system for cancer care. *Wireless Networks*: 1–16.

33 Parra, S., Carranza, E., Coole, J. et al. (2020). Development of low-cost point-of-care technologies for cervical cancer prevention based on a single-board computer. *IEEE Journal of Translational Engineering in Health and Medicine's* 8: 1–10.

34 Kurniawan, A. (2019). Introduction to raspberry pi. In: *Raspbian OS Programming with the Raspberry Pi*, 1–25. Springer.

35 Pajankar, A. (2017). Introduction to single board computers and raspberry pi. In: *Raspberry Pi Image Processing Programming*, 1–24. Springer.

36 Upton, E. (2016). Raspberry pi 2 on sale now at $35. *Raspberry Pi.*

37 Raspberry Pi (2015). Raspberry pi 3 model b. *online]*.(www.raspberrypi.org).

38 Shilpashree, K.S., Lokesha, H., and Shivkumar, H. (2015). Implementation of image processing on raspberry pi. International Journal of Advanced Research in Computer and Communication. *Engineering* 4 (5): 199–202.

39 Reebs, S.R. (1998). Ultrasonic sensor, November 22 1988. US Patent 4,785,664.

40 Yulianto, A. et al. (2019). Design prototype of audio guidance system for blind by using raspberry pi and fuzzy logic controller. In: *Journal of Physics: Conference Series*, vol. 1230, 012024. IOP Publishing.

41 Paras Doshi, Yash Shirke, Tejas Hegde, and Pranav Dhanvij. (2018). Text reader for visually impaired using google cloud vision api, 4 (12): 2349–6002.

42 Beutel, J., Sonka, M., Kundel, H.L. et al. (eds.) (2000). *Handbook of Medical Imaging: Medical Image Processing and Analysis 2*. SPIE Press.

43 Sonka, M., Hlavac, V., and Boyle, R. (1993). Image pre-processing. In: *Image Processing, Analysis and Machine Vision*, 56–111. Springer.

44 Pham, D.L., Chenyang, X., and Prince, J.L. (2000). Current methods in medical image segmentation. *Annual Review of Biomedical Engineering* 2 (1): 315–337.

45 Sharma, N. and Aggarwal, L.M. (2010). Automated medical image segmentation techniques. *Journal of Medical Physics* 35 (1): 3.

46 Pohle, R. and Toennies, K.D. (2001). Segmentation of medical images using adaptive region growing. In: *Medical Imaging 2001: Image Processing*, vol. 4322, 1337–1346. International Society for Optics and Photonics.

47 Bai, B., Liu, P.-Z., Yong-Zhao, D., and Luo, Y.-M. (2018). Automatic segmentation of cervical region in colposcopic images using K-means. *Australasian Physical & Engineering Sciences in Medicine* 41 (4): 1077–1085.

48 Lange, H. (2005). Automatic detection of multi-level acetowhite regions in rgb color images of the uterine cervix. In: *Medical Imaging 2005: Image Processing*, vol. 5747, 1004 1017. International Society for Optics and Photonics.

49 Mariarputham, E.J. and Stephen, A. (2015). Nominated texture based cervical cancer classification. *Computational and Mathematical Methods in Medicine* 2015.

50 Jusman, Y., Ng, S.C., and Osman, N.A.A. (2014). Intelligent screening systems for cervical cancer. *The Scientific World Journal* 2014.

51 Gómez-Mayorga, M.E., Gallegos-Funes, F.J., De-la Rosa-Vázquez, J.M. et al. (2009). Diagnosis of cervical cancer using the median M-type radial basis function (MMRBF) neural network. In: *Mexican International Conference on Artificial Intelligence*, 258–267. Springer.

52 Li, Z. and Najarian, K. (2001). Automated classification of Pap smear tests using neural networks. In: *IJCNN'01. International Joint Conference on Neural Networks. Proceedings (Cat. No. 01CH37222)*, vol. 4, 2899–2901. IEEE.

53 Mat-Isa, N.A., Mashor, M.Y., and Othman, N.H. (2008). An automated cervical pre-cancerous diagnostic system. *Artificial Intelligence in Medicine* 42 (1): 1–11.

54 Thiran, J.-P. and Macq, B. (1996). Morphological feature extraction for the classification of digital images of cancerous tissues. *IEEE Transactions on Biomedical Engineering* 43 (10): 1011–1020.

55 Arya, M., Mittal, N., and Singh, G. (2018). Texture-based feature extraction of smear images for the detection of cervical cancer. *IET Computer Vision* 12 (8): 1049–1059.

56 Ji, Q., Engel, J., and Craine, E. (2000). Texture analysis for classification of cervix lesions. *IEEE Transactions on Medical Imaging* 19 (11): 1144–1149.

57 Sneha, K., Arunvinodh, C. et al. (2016). Cervical cancer detection and classification using texture analysis. *Biomedical and Pharmacology Journal* 9 (2): 663–671.

58 Wei, L., Gan, Q., and Ji, T. (2017). Cervical cancer histology image identification method based on texture and lesion area features. *Computer Assisted Surgery* 22 (sup1): 186–199.

59 Suryatenggara, J., Ane, B.K., Pandjaitan, M., and Steinberg, W. (2009). Pattern recognition on 2d cervical cytological digital images for early detection of cervix cancer. In: *2009 World Congress on Nature & Biologically Inspired Computing (NaBIC)*, 257–262. IEEE.

60 Van Raad, V. (2005). Image analysis and segmentation of anatomical features of cervix uteri in color space. In: *2005 13th European Signal Processing Conference*, 1–4. IEEE.

61 Ashok, B. and Aruna, P. (2016). Comparison of feature selection methods for diagnosis of cervical cancer using SVM classifier. *International Journal of Engineering Research and Applications* 6: 94–99.

62 Hallinan, J. (2001). Feature selection and classification in the diagnosis of cervical cancer. *The Practical Handbook of Genetic Algorithms Applications*: 167–202.

63 Iliyasu, A.M. and Fatichah, C. (2017). A quantum hybrid PSO combined with fuzzy k-NN approach to feature selection and cell classification in cervical cancer detection. *Sensors* 17 (12): 2935.

64 Jiayi, L., Song, E., Ghoneim, A., and Alrashoud, M. (2020). Machine learning for assisting cervical cancer diagnosis: an ensemble approach. *Future Generation Computer Systems* 106: 199–205.

65 Hu, Z., Tang, J., Wang, Z. et al. (2018). Deep learning for image-based cancer detection and diagnosis- a survey. *Pattern Recognition* 83: 134–149.

66 World Health Organization (WHO) et al. (2015). Cervical cancer prevention and control saves lives in the republic of korea. Diakses di http://www.who.int/news-room/feature-stories/detail/cervical-cancerprevention-and-control-saves-lives-in-the-republic-of-korea [diakses 30 April 2018].

9

A Multi-Domain Perspective of Future Directions for VANETs for Emergency Message Dissemination

Ravneet Kaur[1,2], Ramkumar Ketti Ramachandran[2], Robin Doss[1], and Lei Pan[1]

[1] *School of Information Technology, Deakin University, Victoria, Geelong, Australia*
[2] *Chitkara University Institute of Engineering and Technology, Chitkara University, Punjab, Rapura, India*

9.1 Introduction

The term "vehicular communication" was first coined in 1999 by Klaus Eitzenberger to attain safety, traffic control, dynamic navigation aids, and the mobile office. This invention was related to the centralized approach where computers were performing network applications, transmission, reception, recording, or processing data between vehicles, according to Sun et al. [1]. Later on, the concept of distributed message communication came into existence. According to Briesemeister and Hommel [2], radio communications effectively enable the distributed message dissemination strategy in vehicles. However, Xu et al. [3] studied the feasibility for vehicle safety messages in dedicated short range communication (DSRC) and analyzed the memory-less channel modeling. IEEE 802.11p with DSRC followed a WAVE architecture for communication between roadside unit (RSU) and on-board unit (OBU). The WAVE (wireless access in vehicle environment) architecture uses 27 Mbps of data rate with a 5.9 GHz frequency range. The IEEE 802.11p standard plays a vital role in vehicular ad hoc networks (VANETs).

Considering the safety applications, the focus of the automobile industry has been diverted to electronic technologies. The car industry has installed collision detection sensors and electronic control units (ECUs) for making transportation intelligent. Besides, the research community has provided

IoT-Enabled Smart Healthcare Systems, Services and Applications, First Edition.
Edited by Shalli Rani, Maheswar Rajagopal, Neeraj Kumar and Syed Hassan Ahmed Shah.

various solutions for addressing road fatalities, communication range, message delivery, rapid topology change, and mobility pattern. Other issues such as channel modeling, bandwidth wastage, and repetitive message broadcasting to the nodes are prominent. Thus, a suitable emergency message dissemination strategy is applied to the healthcare services, police, and other related infrastructure for immediate help.

This chapter discusses emergency message dissemination in vehicular environments. We consider the multi-domain perspective of the emergency message dissemination regarding the reactive response toward a road fatality in various traffic scenarios. This emergency notification is flagged to the nearby hospitals, pharmacies, and other infrastructure in the VANET. We chose to focus on the role of VANETs with Internet of Things (IoT), fog computing, and blockchain for the healthcare system. Thus, most recent technologies and future trends represent state-of-the-art solutions and build the framework for vehicular communications to deal with emergencies.

The chapter is organized as follows:

- We start with a general discussion on the various trends of technologies with VANETs to serve the emergency message dissemination in Section 9.2. In this part, we will provide the overview and the applications of the IoT, fog computing, and blockchain with VANETs.
- In Section 9.3, we discuss a few questions: What is the role of VANETs in healthcare? How will these advanced technologies and trends benefit the healthcare systems with VANETs? This section explains in detail the most recently proposed solutions for the fast delivery of emergency messages and maximum coverage and includes a case study.
- Our novel research proposal is presented in Section 9.4 by highlighting clustering in multi-domain VANETs emergency message dissemination for the healthcare system.
- The current facilities provided in simulators, testbeds, and interfaces are discussed in Section 9.5. Limitations of the current system and scope of emergency message dissemination in VANETs are also explained.
- We discuss the upcoming trends and possible directions for emergency message dissemination in VANETs along with health care system.
- Section 9.7 provides the conclusion for this chapter.

9.2 Future Directions of Multi-Domain VANETs Emergency Message Dissemination

In VANETs, vehicles are treated as mobile nodes and are equipped with OBUs and ECUs. These resources are useful for disseminating messages during emergencies. In principle, there are three VANET dissemination

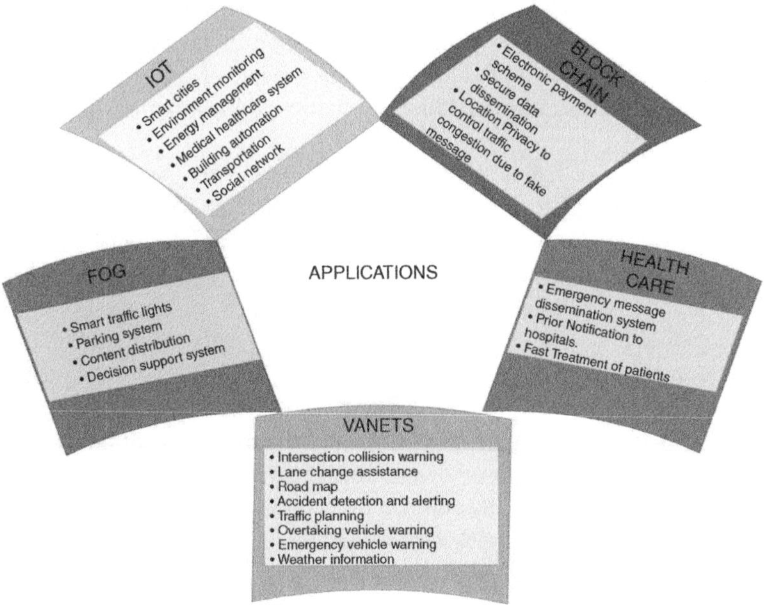

Figure 9.1 Applications are defined. There are five text documents that explain various applications of VANETs with (a) Internet of Things (IOT), (b) blockchain, (c) healthcare, (d) VANETS, and (e) fog computing.

strategies, namely (i) pull, (ii) push, and (iii) hybrid. The "push down" strategy is favorable for safety applications in VANETs, while the built in units in the vehicles monitor environmental conditions and disseminate messages. For the successful and appropriate traversing of the message, traveling path, traveling time, and traveling mode are the crucial factors. With the increase in traffic, road congestion is another issue. To solve these traffic-related issues and saving human lives, Varun Chand and Karthikeyan [4] listed several available technologies. Figure 9.1 presents the applications of the multi-domain behavior of VANETs.

The following subsection describes various technologies in trend with VANETs.

9.2.1 Relationship of VANETs with IoT, Blockchain, and Fog Computing

Internet of Things (IoT) is a computing concept that connects the devices embedded with electronics, sensors, and actuators. It builds the network by enabling physical devices such as vehicles and homes to exchange data. Three networks are formed when IoT is combined with vehicles—inter-vehicle network, intra-vehicle network, and vehicular mobile Internet. These three network types support various applications, including smart cities, environment management, energy management, medical healthcare system, building automation, transportation, and social networking [4].

The limitation of IoT is the storage of electronic devices. To fulfill the emergency message dissemination requirement, vehicles require other technologies. A solution to process data is sending data through the cloud but this presents issues such as lack of mobility support and high-end to end delay. Hence, fog computing has been proposed to overcome these shortcomings [5].

Fog computing with VANETs is a promising approach to overcome the delay in a decentralized network and optimize the bandwidth usage, thus named vehicular fog computing. Fog computing provides decentralization to all the nodes and reduces overhead on the core network layer. These nodes are distributed geographically and hence create a layer, names fog computing layer. While communicating with the fog computing layer, vehicles act as fog computing nodes and fog computing users according to the service required. When the vehicles are parked or in traffic jams, they act as fog computing nodes and have minimum storage capacity due to flooding of message communication however, posses high efficiency and low latency [5].

This approach leads to offload the RSUs tasks, autonomous driving, video crowdsourcing, content distribution, smart traffic light, and decision support system [6]. For example, during the event-driven applications, the RSU contributes by investigating the free parking slot for the emergency vehicle. Similarly, a smart traffic light system plays a vital role by sensing the autonomous vehicle driving toward hospitals and thus supports the healthcare system.

The major drawback of fog computing with VANETs is a high end-to-end delay, high bandwidth usage, weak security, and poor reliability. More research is needed in this domain for applications that are more time sensitive. Though this approach is useful for quickly saving the patient records, it should be done securely.

Blockchain with VANETs is the emerging research area that provides a secure, authenticated, and trusted environment for V2X (vehicle-to-everything) communication. It is pertinent to facilitate recording and tracking resources with a centralized computing platform. Blockchain maintains a ledger for event message exchange to avoid collateral damage. There are various advantages of using blockchain with VANETs such as secure data, location privacy to control traffic congestion due to fake messages, non-repudiation, transparency, and electronic payment scheme [7]. While

Table 9.1 Limitations of VANETs with (a) IoT being an IoV, (b) fog computing being a vehicular fog computing network, and (c) blockchain.

IoT	Fog computing	Blockchain
low storage capacity	more end-to-end delay	low capacity
security	high bandwidth usage	increased overhead
technology over-reliance	security	increased verification time
	reliability	high deployment cost

communicating messages from one vehicle to another or to infrastructure, the data message is divided into block segments. Once the block is added to the chain, the data block cannot be modified. For any update or modification in the block, smart contracts will be used.

Blockchain with VANETs has slow data storage, long overhead, and long verification time, which affect the system's performance, increase deployment cost, and limit scalability [8].

Table 9.1 lists the limitations of VANETs with IoT, Fog Computing, and Blockchain.

9.3 Role of VANETs in Healthcare Systems

The increased number of deaths due to overcrowded roads and traffic mismanagement opens various research and development opportunities in VANETs. The development in e-health services and smart mobility ease the elder person checkups. The deployment of wireless e-health services and on-time delivery of reliable medication prompts the healthcare stakeholders. The growing demand of VANETs within healthcare provides various benefits and open challenges to the community that is significantly different from the random topology change or mobility patterns of VANETs [9].

Another advancement in VANETs within healthcare is telemedicine to develop smart healthcare systems in rural and urban areas. This mobile solution supports developing countries such as India, where building the physical structures is quite tricky. This consultation is more feasible and cost effective as it reduces medical costs, travel expenses, and time. Such solutions are especially useful during pandemics and for the people who live in rural areas [10].

As shown in Figure 9.2, during emergency message dissemination, any technology in IoT, fog computing, and blockchain can provide useful

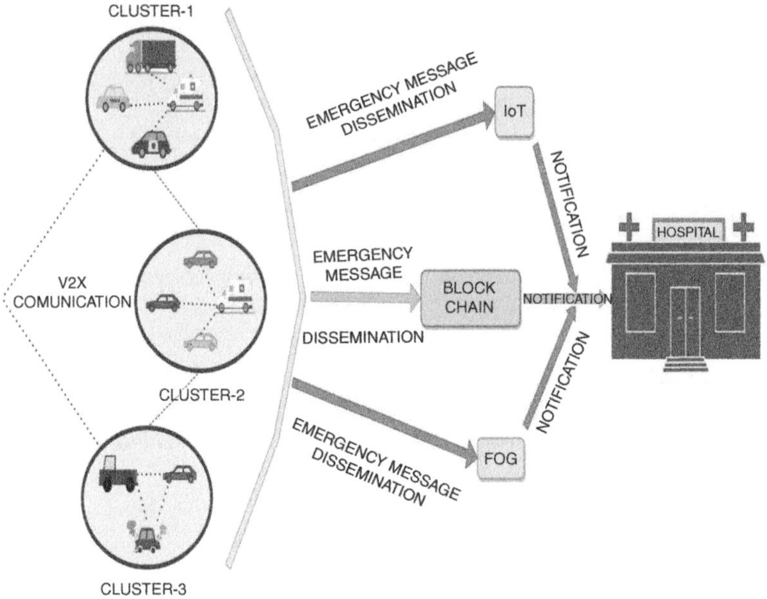

Figure 9.2 Diagrammatic representation of multi-domain future perspective of emergency message dissemination in VANETs for healthcare system.

information to the appropriate infrastructure. However, the clustering framework improves communication by providing the opportunity for full connectivity and maximum coverage. The responsibility of data packet sharing is distributed to all other nodes and thus balances the load. This setup facilitates fast communication. The collaboration of connected vehicles helps implement real-time applications. In particular, several routing protocols and frameworks are presented in Kaur et al. [11].

In Section 9.3.1, a case study is presented to show how the emergency message dissemination notification is effective in a real-time environment.

9.3.1 Case Study

When a serious traffic accident happens, the time taken by the emergency services to arrive is crucial. Most deaths during accidents happen due to the unavailability of emergency services. According to the World Health Organization (WHO), by 2030, road fatalities will be the seventh leading cause of death worldwide. To reduce road accidents, the knowledge of the road events such as congested roads, notification of road fatality, or other emergencies plays a crucial role. For example, the notification of road accidents will notify the associated personals such as hospitals, pharmacies, and the police so as to reduce the delay in providing emergency aid.

Perhaps that will be the automobile industry's future, where vehicles talk to one another and with the infrastructure. Currently, the US Department of Transportation (DoT) is working on connected vehicles. Even that would greatly impact this pandemic where in developing countries such as India, people need E-permits to enter another state.

VANETs provide an opportunity to cover large areas using clustering, in which the cluster head (CH) is selected to pass the emergency message to all the vehicles timely, as shown in Figure 9.2. They will help control the traffic flow and reduce the resulting congestion at accident sites. This arrangement will drastically reduce road fatalities, save human lives, reduce fuel consumption, and save drivers' money, ultimately making our transportation safer and smarter.

Different techniques can be used to quickly disseminate emergency messages to support the healthcare system. Section 9.4 elaborates on various technologies.

9.4 Techniques Used for Fast Delivery of Emergency Message in VANETs to Help the Healthcare System

Launching an intelligent transportation system (ITS) is a way to provide managed and controlled traffic on the road. This will make use of smart, safe, and synchronized ways of transportation. There is a tremendous increase in the number of vehicles that leads to traffic congestion and traffic accidents. During such emergencies, there is a need to communicate the event information to the nearby vehicles, hospitals, pharmacies, police, and many more. There is a possibility that all vehicles would not receive the emergency information due to their rapid topology change or they would not lie in the communication range. Thus, there is a need to ensure the full connectivity of the network and reliable communication. It helps secure the data from intruders, spoofing, denial of service, and many more attacks. According to Kaur et al. [11], clustering is the solution for such problems. Clustering plays an instrumental role in providing the maximum coverage by selecting the most relevant CH selection parameters. When integrated with various technologies in ITS, this framework will act as a support for the healthcare system.

The following subsections describe recent technologies to facilitate emergency situations.

9.4.1 Role of Clustering in VANETs for Healthcare System

When vehicles are moving on the road, the CH is selected as the group head. The group members and their neighboring nodes' positions can be identified by the hardware components and system controller modules. By knowing the position ID, location ID, and other parameters, a realistic setup can be established to optimize the road traffic.

Whenever there is a road accident, to avoid traffic jams, congestion on the road, and facilitate immediate first aid, a structure is needed to broadcast all the information in the vicinity. Communicating such sensitive information is a crucial task because there are chances of spoofing. Hence, an attacker may change the information. Another issue is the link breakage due to rapid topology change. The mobile nature of VANETs has different patterns of movement. Thus, there is a need for a full-connectivity structure to disseminate emergency messages. One of the most prominent solutions is clustering [11]. Using the appropriate framework for delivering messages to the RSUs and other infrastructure, vehicles can communicate within the specified range. If the vehicles are out of range, clustering is the solution. In clustering, CH selection is based on metric selection. The selection of metrics is application-specific. If there is an emergency event, then time is the most important parameter. If there is retrieving of patients' data, then clustering with privacy preservation is the suitable approach.

Another critical parameter is the traffic scenario. The selection of parameters also depends on the sparse and dense traffic scenario. If there are less vehicles and are far from each other, link breakage is the problem. If jammed vehicles caused traffic congestion, bandwidth wastage and increased overhead become the challenge. Thus, various optimized clustering techniques are provided to deal with the real challenges of VANETs. However, very little work has been done on the role of clustering in VANETs with healthcare. There is a wide scope of the role of clustering in the healthcare system. Other advantages of the clustering in VANETs with healthcare are listed below.

- Maximum coverage area;
- Reduced bandwidth wastage;
- Low link breakage;
- Backup support for transmitting messages;
- Ability of secure message dissemination;
- Treatment started before arriving to the hospital;
- Hospital arrangements made beforehand; and
- Online medical consultation is provided as an alternative option for elderly and rural people.

However, network congestion often occurs in high-density areas associated with issues such as flooding, broadcast storm, channel modeling, and security.

9.4.2 Role of Clustering in VANETs with IoT for Healthcare System

The development of IoT with VANETs enhances the commercial interest in healthcare management. The Internet of Vehicle (IoV) [12] is helpful in monitoring the health of patients and maintaining the records. Various architectures and communication protocols have been proposed to update the status of patients regularly. This type of solution acts as a possibility of rescue for the patients during emergencies. Another possible use case is road fatalities. If the communication quickly reaches the nearby hospital or broadcasted within the vicinity, , the injured could have been saved. The following are the advantages of IoV.

- Providing emergency aid during peak hours;
- Time management;
- Prior knowledge to a nearby hospital;
- Emergency notification to police;
- Emergency notification to ambulance service; and
- Traffic management.

Besides, there are various limitations such as bandwidth wastage, link breakage, intruder attack, connectivity issues, coverage area, unreliable network connectivity, resource utilization, and broadcast storm. Thus, clustering plays a vital role in IoV. From the above discussion, it can be concluded that there are various applications in IoV that need to be explored. Working with sensors and collecting information from the environment help predict the real-time expenses of deploying the VANET systems during transportation to reduce the waste and increase efficiency [13].

9.4.3 Role of Clustering in VANETs with Fog Computing for Healthcare System

Nowadays, much interest has been driven to the VANETs and fog computing. According to Popescu et al. [14], various fog Computing architectures are proposed. Fog computing nodes act as RSUs and are responsible for group formation to ensure message dissemination to the complete network and provide secure route services. RSUs can be deployed on the fog computing nodes, and data processing is the extended feature. Fog computing nodes' distributed control at different geographic locations is responsible for mobile communication, whereas the centralized control is for static communication. Having the group head as a fog computing node in a small area acts as a small hub of reports and online treatment directory for patients [14]. All the records with comparison metrics could be available to the healthcare workers to treat the patients. Thus, fog computing nodes will act as a repository while the patient is in an emergency. The following are the advantages of fog computing:

- Backup storage is available;
- Distributed structure provides fast access to patients' data;
- It's cost effective;
- Latency reduction; and
- Enhanced compliance.

However, various issues exist in vehicular fog computing, including unpredictable trajectory, scalability, mobility of vehicles, frequent interruptions, link breakage, malicious vehicle joining, network flooded by irrelevant data, chances of data modification, reliability, and security of the network [15].

9.4.4 Role of Clustering in VANETs with Blockchain for Healthcare System

Various secure protocols have been proposed considering the trust factor. During the retrieval of distributed data from different geographic locations, locations act as unique clusters. The data can be traversed through blocks at the time of emergency. Thus, sensitive data is shared in the hospital vicinity. These records are distributed in various hospitals defined under a unique ID to retrieve the previous consultation. These records are generally called electronic medical records (EMR). For accessing these records in a secure manner, blockchain plays a crucial role [16].

With numerous applications in blockchain with VANETs, the technical implementation lacks a data-sharing and -management system and thus is unable to maintain traceability [7]. When data flow happens during an emergency, there is a need for storage space. This will increase the bloating problem. The rapid topology change and mobility of nodes make proof-of-work (PoW) difficult by having a limited time for exchanging information blocks. This information exchange depends on the trust factor. Once the nodes are verified, the information exchange happens. The mobile nature of nodes cannot provide an accurate analysis of nodes that can participate in block propagation.

Various solutions are provided in Kim [17] such as security and credibility, real identity versus public keys, smart contracts with VANETs, and energy contributions. However, the impact of mobility on nodes and its metrics are not addressed for blockchain performance. Nevertheless, blockchain does not fully support VANETs. Thus, other challenges include the addition of blocks and exchange of blocks in mobile nodes of a blockchain system. The following are the various advantages where blockchain is used in VANETs [18]:

- Collect sensor data;
- Broadcast signatures to surrounding vehicles;
- Verify incoming signatures;
- Preventing forged data;
- Mutual authentication with reduced dependency on certificate;
- Authority;
- Scalability;
- Privacy protection;
- Message confidentiality, integrity, and non-repudiation; and
- Speedy revocation without additional overhead.

9.4.5 Implications of Multi-Domain Perspective of VANETs for Emergency Message Dissemination

In this chapter, we have discussed various technologies, including IoT, Fog Computing, and Blockchain with respect to VANETs and the role of emergency message dissemination using those technologies in the healthcare system. However, we concluded that a particular combined structure needs to be proposed for benefiting the healthcare community and the public. Figure 9.3 shows the diagrammatic representation of the multi-domain future perspective of VANETs. This figure explains the two following aspects:

- The rectangular shape blocks are defining the individual contribution of their technology in VANETs. For example, vehicles are embedded with IoT devices and perform operations after sensing the environment as needed. Similarly, fog computing helps provide storage capacity in geographical locations and within the vicinity thus providing fast and timely delivery of messages.
- The second way of proposing the structure is application-specific. For example, if there is a road accident, IoT devices sense the environment such as number of vehicles, infrastructure, speed of vehicle, directions etc to perform clustering and hence sends the emergency notification. This

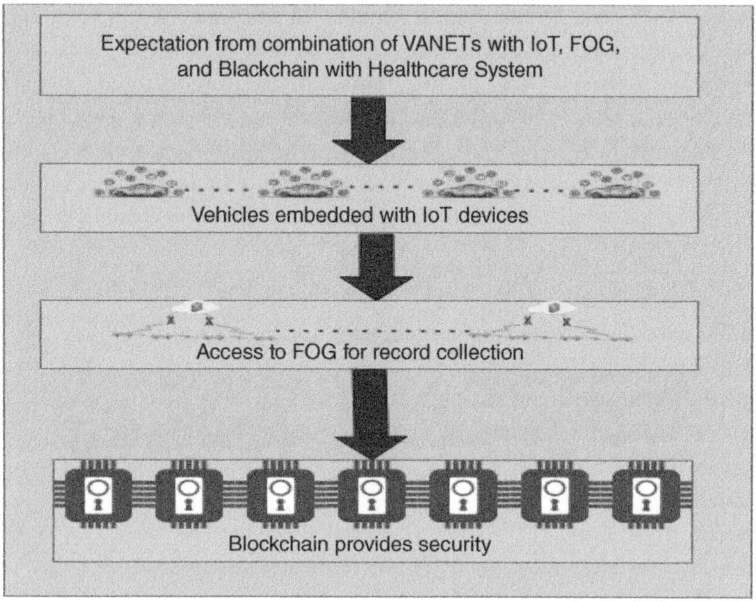

Figure 9.3 Diagrammatic representation of multi-domain future perspective of emergency message dissemination in VANETs.

notification can be sent to the nearby crowd to check the availability of a doctor or the pharmacy; thus, it could provide immediate first aid.

- The hospital would have time to collect the treatment data of the patient beforehand. Fog computing plays a crucial role to transfer the data securely, and blockchain comes into the picture.

From the above discussion, it can be concluded that various research domains are open for research.

9.5 Current Facilities and Limitations for Implementing the Real-Time Environment

VANET is the most promising research area and offers various safety applications. Because of vehicles' unpredictable movement and rapid topology change, the automobile industry is working in the direction of smart transportation. In 2006, the US DoT had identified eight warning notifications in which vehicles were communicating with roadside equipment (RSE). To evaluate the proposed work and predict the VANET system's performance, it is costly to establish a new setup or work in a real-time environment. Thus, network simulators, traffic simulators, and testbeds are used to analyze the proposed work before market launch [19]. The following is the discussion on this testing content.

- There are four models: (i) traffic model, which defines the mobility pattern in three classes: microscopic, macroscopic, and mesoscopic; (ii) driver and vehicle model, in which the driver's behavior (how the driver responds during an emergency or after receiving the emergency notification) is important; (iii) communication model, which defines the different routing strategies and communication environment; and (iv) the application model, which is the scenario and application-specific model.
- Simulators: There are two types of simulators required to implement any scenario: (i) traffic simulator, and (ii) network simulator. The traffic simulators include Simulation of Urban Mobility (SUMO) and VISSIM (Verker In Stadten Simulation Model). These traffic simulators possess various features that can be modeled as needed. However, the network simulators such as NS2, NS3, OMNET++ (Objective Modular Network Testbed in C++), and VEINS (Vehicles in Network Simulation) possess comprehensive network routing protocols. These simulators are useful in implementing and then verifying the results according to the proposed ideas to solve the designated issue [20].
- Testbeds: They are also known as field operating testing. Although VANETs can be implemented in various simulators, realistic field operations are lacking. Due to the high cost of establishing such an environment, the US DoT and Florida DoT provide testbeds. One needs to book the slot and test the proposed algorithm to obtain the actual results [21].

9.6 Discussion on Upcoming Trends and Possibilities with Future Readings

Upcoming ITS integrated with multi-domain technologies will offer a revolution toward global automation, the response to emergency situations, and human safety. Different techniques have been explored in this chapter. The IEEE, Florida DoT, and National Highway Traffic Safety Administration (NHTSA) which is part of the US DoT are the leading bodies for providing funds for innovations in ITS. As shown in Figure 9.4, various research challenges are identified to support VANETs with the healthcare system. These

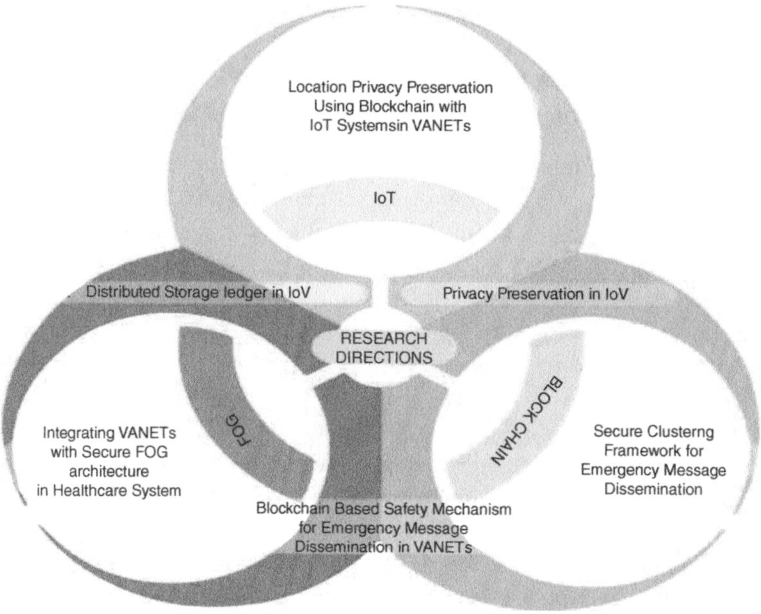

Figure 9.4 Emerging research directions in VANETs with multi-domain perspective for emergency message dissemination.

research directions need further research and investigation. The open research areas are listed below.

- The scope of VANETs with blockchain is the most prominent research area. Researchers can explore this combination and benefit the research community in terms of publications, future directions, security, and many more [8].
- For dissertations, VANETs with IoT will be helpful. One can embed the electronic devices and check the real-time applications. This domain provides good opportunities for start-ups [15].
- Network congestion control is the research area where overloading and bandwidth wastage is the major issue. Thus, data congestion during emergency message dissemination is a prominent domain [22].
- Realistic channel modeling is another challenging metric that needs further attention and is open for research [11].
- For providing the multi-channel data flow in terms of patient records during an emergency, fog computing with blockchain is an emerging trend.

This combination will provide the secured record ledger for traveling of information [6].

International workshops, summits, industrial events, testbeds, and conferences are provided for delivering transportation solutions. We have divided this discussion into four aspects: (i) industrial events, (ii) testbeds, (iii) conferences, and (iv) summits.

- Industrial workshops: MOVE: Mobility Re-imagined is the world's most important mobility event, which provides an opportunity to collaborate and bring the needed change. This event is in its third year and is focused on companies' CEOs and founders. This is a platform for start-ups, innovative solutions, and partnerships that are dedicated to tech and transportation.[a]
- Testbeds: Connecting vehicles in a real-time environment promotes the development and deployment of networked transportation in the automobile industry. The connected vehicles testbed by the US DoT is available for developers to test the technology in a real-time environment through a wireless connection. This testbed provides 5.9 GHz of DSRC to communicate where RSE is embedded. This is the surface where users can test advancements in software and hardware of connected vehicles.[b]
- Conferences: There are various conferences and journals to start reading. The best way to understand any research domain is to identify the difference between surveys, reviews, journals, transactions, and conferences. The upcoming IEEE Vehicular Technology Conference is a highly cited conference whereas IEEE Transactions on ITS is a highly recommended journal to read and publish work. This is a flagship conference hosted by IEEE Vehicular Technology Society under the supervision of J.R. Cruz, Vice President of Conferences.[c]
- Summits: In the year 2021, various summits are lined up. Voice of Car is the Silicon Valley summit to focus on the intersection of voice technology in cars. The vision of the summit is to have a look at the future connected cars and incorporating voice communication by leading automobile manufacturers.[d]

Considering the research community, in continuation with international workshops on OMNET++, the 7th OMNET++ Community Summit was organized in 2020. This summit provided lively discussions, keynotes, tutorials, and ongoing demonstrations to the researchers and helped them to sort various implementation-related issues that occurred during their research. The focus is to bring all the OMNET++ developers and tools together with novel ideas in network simulators.[e]

9.7 Conclusion

In this chapter, we provide the role of VANETs in healthcare from a multi-domain perspective. The effectiveness and need of IoT, fog computing, and blockchain with VANETs give the upcoming researchers a new direction. Overseeing the traditional VANET structure, we observe the emerging trend and the broad scope of VANETs in healthcare systems. Beyond various safety and non-safety applications in VANETs, we present a case study and its implications in multiple crucial factors, including full connectivity, maximum coverage area, and scalability. We argue that clustering is a promising approach for achieving excellent results for emergency message dissemination. The future trends include readings, summits, workshops, and conferences in VANETs.

Notes

a https://www.terrapinn.com/exhibition/move/index.stm.
b https://www.its.dot.gov/research_archives/connected_vehicle/dot_cvbrochure.htm
c https://events.vtsociety.org/vtc2021-spring/about
d https://www.prnewswire.com/news-releases/voice-of-the-car-summit-april-7-8-2020-in-the-silicon-valley-to-focus-on-the-intersection-of-voice-technology-and-the-modern-connected-car-301005955.html
e https://summit.omnetpp.org/2020/index.html

Author Biography

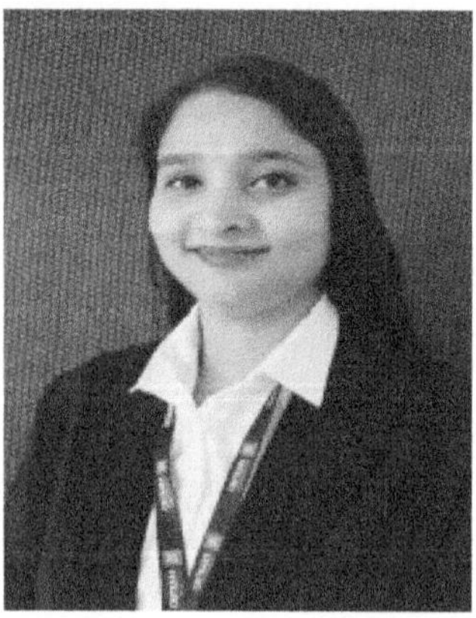

Ravneet Kaur is a student of higher degree by research at Deakin University, Geelong, Australia, with the Research Partner Department of Computer Science and Engineering, Chitkara University Institute of Engineering and Technology, Chitkara University, Punjab, India, under Deakin India Research Initiative (DIRI) programme.

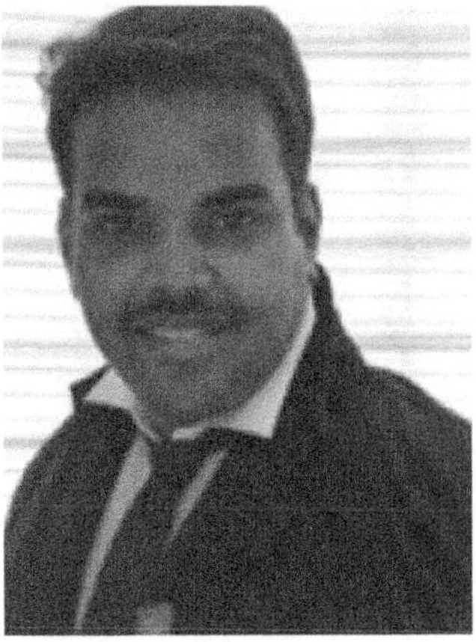

Dr. K.R. Ramkumar is PhD in computer science and engineering from Anna University, Chennai, India, having 17 years of teaching and research experience. He is currently working as an associate professor, Chitkara University Institute of Engineering and Technology, Chitkara University, Punjab, India. His areas of expertise are network security, key management, and relational database management systems in advancement. His research includes solving the routing issues, dealing with security and node failure apprehensions of wireless sensor networks. Much of his work has been on improving the understanding, design and performance analysis of different routing and security algorithms of Wireless Sensor Networks (WSN). He is also working with the Extensible Markup Language (XML) and resolving the data integrity and consistency issues on web communications.

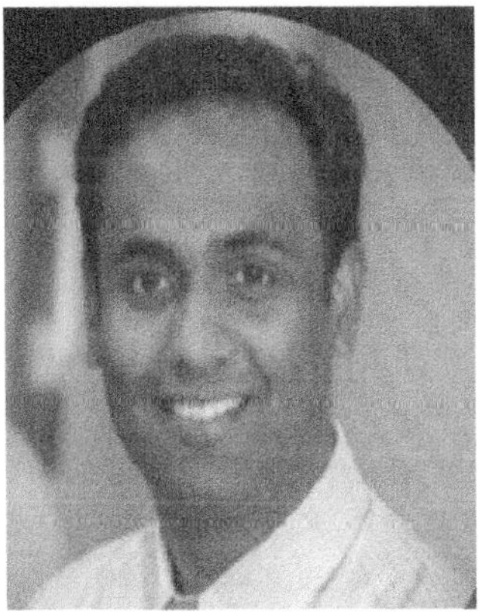

Prof. Robin Doss is a professor of information technology and the Deputy Head of the School of Information Technology. Robin leads the Internet of Things (IoT) and Cyber Physical Systems (CPS) security program at the Deakin Centre for Cyber Security Research and Innovation (CSRI) and is the Co-Director of the IoT research cluster at Deakin. He is a senior member of the IEEE.

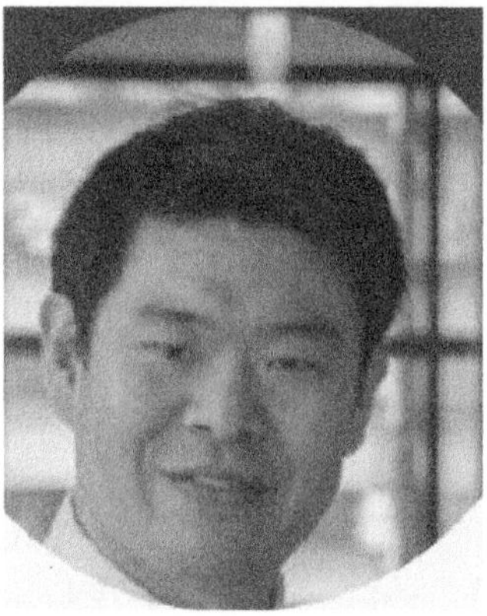

Dr. Lei Pan received his PhD in computer forensics from Deakin University, Australia, in 2008. He is currently a senior lecturer with the School of Information Technology, Deakin University. His research interests are cyber security and IoT. He has authored 50+ research papers in refereed international journals and conferences.

References

1 Sun, M.-t., Feng, W.-c., and Ten-Hwang, L. (2000. ISSN 1090-3038. adoi: https://doi.org/10.1109/VETECF.2000.886811). GPS-based message broadcast for adaptive inter-vehicle communications. In: *Vehicular Technology Conference Fall 2000. IEEE VTS Fall VTC2000. 52nd Vehicular Technology Conference (Cat. No.00CH37152)*, vol. 6, 2685–2692. URL http://ieeexplore.ieee.org/lpdocs/epic03/wrapper.htm?arnumber=886811.

2 Briesemeister, L. and Hommel, G. (2000). Role-based multicast in highly mobile but sparsely connected ad hoc networks. In: *2000 1st Annual Workshop on Mobile and Ad Hoc Networking and Computing, MobiHOC 2000*, 45–50. https://doi.org/10.1109/MOBHOC.2000.869212.

3 Xu, Q., Mak, T., Ko, J., and Sengupta, R. (2004. ISSN 09609822. doi: https://doi.org/10.1145/1023875.1023879). Vehicle-to-vehicle safety messaging in DSRC. In: *Proceedings of the First ACM Workshop on Vehicular Ad Hoc Networks - VANET '04*, page 19. URL http://portal.acm.org/citation.cfm?doid=1023875.1023879.

4 Varun Chand, H. and Karthikeyan, J. (2018). Survey on the role of iot in intelligent transportation system. *Indonesian Journal of Electrical Engineering and Computer Science* 110 (3): 936–941.

5 Mekki, T., Jabri, I., Chaari, L., and Rachedi, A. (2020). A survey on vehicular fog computing: motivation, architectures, taxonomy, and issues. In: *Workshops of the International Conference on Advanced Information Networking and Applications*, 159–168. Springer.

6 Lai, Y., Yang, F., Zhang, L., and Lin, Z. (2018). Distributed public vehicle system based on fog nodes and vehicular sensing. *IEEE Access* 6: 22011–22024.

7 Tariq, F., Anwar, M., Janjua, A.R. et al. (2020). Blockchain in wsns, vanets, iots and healthcare: a survey. In: *Workshops of the International Conference on Advanced Information Networking and Applications*, 267–279. Springer.

8 Lu, Z., Liu, W., Wang, Q. et al. (2018). A privacy-preserving trust model based on blockchain for vanets. *IEEE Access* 6: 45655–45664.

9 Bilal, R. and Khan, B.M. (2021). The role of vehicular ad hoc networks in intelligent transport systems for healthcare. In: *Advances in Multidisciplinary Medical Technologies – Engineering, Modeling and Findings* (eds. A. Khelassi and V.V. Estrela), 155–183. Cham: Springer International Publishing. ISBN: 978-3-030-57552-6.

10 Mukhopadhyay, A. (2017). QoS based telemedicine technologies for rural healthcare emergencies. In: *2017 IEEE Global Humanitarian Technology Conference (GHTC)*, 1–7. https://doi.org/10.1109/GHTC.2017.8239296.

11 Kaur, R., Ramachandran, R.K., Doss, R., and Pan, L. (2021). The importance of selecting clustering parameters in vanets: a survey. *Computer Science Review* 40: 100392.

12 Thirugnanam, T. and Ghalib, M.R. (2020). A new healthcare architecture using iov technology for continuous health monitoring system. *Health and Technology* 100 (1): 289–302.

13 Hatim, S.M., Elias, S.J., Awang, N., and Darus, M.Y. (2018). Vanets and internet of things (IoT): a discussion. *Indonesian Journal of Electrical Engineering and Computer Science* 12: 218–224.

14 Popescu, O., Sha-Mohammad, S., Abdel-Wahab, H. et al. (2017). Automatic incident detection in intelligent transportation systems using aggregation of traffic parameters collected through v2i communications. *IEEE Intelligent Transportation Systems Magazine* 90 (2): 64–75.

15 Wang, X., Zha, X., Ni, W. et al. (2019). Survey on blockchain for internet of things. *Computer Communications* 136: 10–29.

16 Alex Blanter and Mark Holman. Internet of things 2020: a glimpse into the future. *Available at Kearney* https://www.atkearney.com/documents/4634214/6398631/AT+Kearney_Internet+of+Things, 2020.

17 Kim, S. (2019). Impacts of mobility on performance of blockchain in vanet. *IEEE Access* 7: 68646–68655.

18 Majumder, S., Mathur, A., and Javaid, A.Y. (2019). A study on recent applications of blockchain technology in vehicular adhoc network (vanet). In: *National Cyber Summit*, 293–308. Springer.

19 Liang, W., Li, Z., Zhang, H. et al. (2015). Vehicular ad hoc networks: architectures, research issues, methodologies, challenges, and trends. *International Journal of Distributed Sensor Networks* 110 (8): 745303.

20 Martinez, F.J., Toh, C.K., Cano, J.-C. et al. (2011). A survey and comparative study of simulators for vehicular ad hoc networks (vanets). *Wireless Communications and Mobile Computing* 110 (7): 813–828.

21 Secinti, G., Canberk, B., Duong, T.Q., and Shu, L. (2017). Software defined architecture for vanet: a testbed implementation with wireless access management. *IEEE Communications Magazine* 550 (7): 135–141.

22 Ali, G.G.M.N., Chan, E., and Li, W. (2014). On scheduling data access with cooperative load balancing in vehicular ad hoc networks (vanets). *The Journal of Supercomputing* 670 (2): 438–468.

Index

IoT-Enabled Smart Healthcare Systems, Services and Applications, First Edition.
Edited by Shalli Rani, Maheswar Rajagopal, Neeraj Kumar and Syed Hassan Ahmed Shah.

f

Printed and bound by CPI Group (UK) Ltd, Croydon, CR0 4YY